Table of Contents

Introduction

Chapter 1: Getting Started with Meal Prep

Chapter 2: Weekly Meal Prep Calendar

- Lentil and Spinach Salad
  - Turkey and Vegetable Lettuce Wraps
  - Mediterranean Tuna Salad
  - Pesto and Veggie Pasta Salad
  - Asian-Inspired Tofu Salad
  - Shrimp and Quinoa Bowl
  - Veggie and Hummus Wrap
  - Cucumber and Tuna Salad
  - Pita Bread and Hummus Plate
  - Spaghetti Squash Primavera
  - Eggplant and Tomato Salad
  - Turkey and Quinoa Stuffed Bell Peppers
  - Tomato and Mozzarella Salad
  - Chicken and Vegetable Kebabs
  - Spinach and Feta Omelette
  - Chicken and Vegetable Stir-Fry
  - Mediterranean Chickpea Wrap
  - ...

13. Dinner Recipes
  - Baked Salmon with Lemon-Dill Sauce
  - Grilled Chicken Breast with Quinoa and Steamed Broccoli
  - Baked Salmon with Roasted Vegetables
  - Lentil and Vegetable Stir-Fry
  - Turkey and Spinach Stuffed Bell Peppers
  - Shrimp and Veggie Stir-Fry
  - Sweet Potato and Black Bean Bowl
  - Teriyaki Tofu and Vegetable Stir-Fry
  - Mediterranean Chickpea Salad
  - Pesto Zucchini Noodles
  - Spaghetti Squash with Marinara Sauce
  - Greek Salad with Grilled Chicken
  - Tuna and White Bean Salad
  - Baked Chicken Thighs with Roasted Vegetables
  - Veggie and Tofu Stir-Fry
  - Caprese Stuffed Portobello Mushrooms
  - Cilantro Lime Shrimp with Quinoa
  - Butternut Squash and Spinach Salad
  - Eggplant Parmesan
  - Asian-Inspired Salmon Bowl

Conclusion
- Final Thoughts and Words of Encouragement

INTRODUCTION

Losing weight is a journey, and it's one that many of us embark on at some point in our lives. Whether it's to improve our health, boost our confidence, or simply feel better in our own skin, the desire to shed those extra pounds is a common one. However, the path to successful weight loss can be daunting, filled with obstacles and temptations that threaten to derail our progress. This is where the concept of meal prep comes into play.

Understanding the Importance of Meal Prep for Weight Loss

Meal prep is not just a trendy term or a passing fad; it's a powerful strategy that can make a world of difference on your weight loss journey. At its core, meal prep involves planning and preparing your meals in advance, ensuring that you have healthy and balanced options readily available when hunger strikes. It's a strategy that empowers you to take control of your diet, make informed choices, and ultimately, achieve your weight loss goals. The importance of meal prep cannot be overstated. It is a practical and sustainable approach to managing your caloric intake, ensuring that you consume the right nutrients in the right portions. By taking the time to plan your meals, you can avoid impulsive, unhealthy food choices that often occur when you're hungry and in a rush. Meal prep sets you up for success by eliminating guesswork and temptation, making it easier to stick to your dietary plan. But meal prep is not just about the physical act of cooking and storing food. It's also about the psychological aspect of weight loss. When you have your meals planned and prepared, you remove the stress of deciding what to eat, which can be a significant source of anxiety for many people struggling with their weight. This reduced decision fatigue allows you to focus your mental energy on other aspects of your life, creating a sense of freedom and control that can be incredibly empowering.

Setting Your Weight Loss Goals

Before diving headfirst into the world of meal prep, it's essential to set clear and achievable weight loss goals. These goals serve as your North Star, guiding your efforts and keeping you motivated throughout your journey. Your goals should be specific, measurable, and realistic. Instead of saying, "I want to lose weight," try something like, "I want to lose 20 pounds in the next six months by eating healthier and exercising regularly." Having concrete goals provides you with a sense of purpose and direction. It allows you to track your progress and celebrate your successes along the way. Consider creating both short-term and long-term goals to keep your motivation levels high. Short-term goals can be achieved in a matter of weeks or months, while long-term goals may take a year or more to reach. These goals act as stepping stones on your path to a healthier you.

Remember that weight loss is not just about the number on the scale; it's also about how you feel, both physically and emotionally. Pay attention to non-scale victories, such as increased energy, better sleep, improved mood, and enhanced self-confidence. These positive changes can be just as, if not more, rewarding than the actual weight loss. As you embark on your weight loss journey through meal prep, keep your goals at the forefront of your mind. Visualize your success, and remind yourself why you started this journey in the first place. Weight loss is not always easy, but with determination, consistency, and the right strategies, you can achieve your goals and experience the transformative power of a healthier lifestyle. In the pursuit of weight loss, meal prep is your trusted companion, guiding you towards a healthier, happier you. It's more than just a practical strategy; it's a mindset shift that empowers you to take control of your dietary choices, reduce stress, and achieve your weight loss goals. By setting clear and realistic objectives, you can stay motivated and measure your progress along the way. As you delve deeper into the world of meal prep, remember that your journey is unique to you. There will be challenges and setbacks, but each one presents an opportunity to learn and grow. Embrace the process, and be kind to yourself. Weight loss is not a sprint; it's a marathon, and with dedication and the right tools, you can reach the finish line.
Throughout this book, we'll explore the fundamentals of meal prep, provide you with a comprehensive meal calendar, and offer a wide range of delicious and nutritious recipes to keep your taste buds satisfied. We'll address various dietary preferences and special considerations to ensure that meal prep works for you, no matter your unique circumstances.So, are you ready to embark on this transformative journey towards a healthier you? With meal prep as your ally, there's no limit to what you can achieve. Let's take the

first step together and embrace the power of meal prep for weight loss. Your healthier, happier future awaits.

Chapter 1
Getting Started with Meal Prep

The Basics of Meal Prepping

Meal prepping is the cornerstone of successful weight loss and healthy eating. It's a simple yet powerful strategy that can transform your relationship with food and help you achieve your dietary goals. At its core, meal prepping involves planning, preparing, and portioning your meals in advance, typically for a week or even a month. In this section, we'll delve into the fundamental aspects of meal prepping, exploring why it's so essential, and how you can get started on this journey toward better health and well-being.

Why Meal Prepping Matters

Imagine a typical weekday morning. You wake up late, rush to get ready for work, and find yourself racing against the clock to make it out the door on time. As you head out, you realize you haven't had breakfast yet. The thought of a nutritious meal is quickly overshadowed by the convenience of grabbing a sugary pastry or a fast-food breakfast sandwich. This scenario is all too familiar to many of us, and it's precisely where meal prepping steps in to save the day. Meal prepping matters because it removes the chaos and unpredictability from your daily eating habits. It empowers you to make thoughtful, health-conscious choices, even when life gets busy. By having pre-prepared meals and snacks on hand, you can wave goodbye to impulsive and unhealthy food decisions. Instead, you'll find yourself reaching for a balanced meal that aligns with your goals, whether they're weight loss, muscle gain, or simply maintaining a healthier lifestyle. One of the key benefits of meal prepping is portion control. When you prepare your meals in advance, you have the opportunity to measure and portion your food carefully. This prevents overeating and ensures that you're consuming the right number of calories for your individual needs.

Portion control is a game-changer when it comes to weight management, and meal prepping puts you in the driver's seat. Moreover, meal prepping can save you time and money in the long run. Yes, it does require an initial investment of time and effort, but the payoff is worth it. Consider the time you spend on a Sunday afternoon preparing meals for the week as an investment in your health and well-being. You'll spend less time in the kitchen on busy weekdays and save money by avoiding costly takeout and restaurant meals.

The Art of Meal Planning

The first step in successful meal prepping is meal planning. This is where you set the stage for the week ahead by deciding what you'll eat and when. The key to effective meal planning is variety and balance. Aim to incorporate a wide range of food groups, including lean proteins, whole grains, fruits, vegetables, and healthy fats, into your meals.

Start by creating a weekly or monthly meal calendar. This calendar will serve as your roadmap, guiding you through your meal prep journey. You can choose to plan all three main meals (breakfast, lunch, and dinner) and snacks, or you can start with one meal at a time. The level of detail in your meal plan is entirely up to you, but the more comprehensive it is, the smoother your meal prepping process will be. When planning your meals, consider your dietary goals and preferences. Are you aiming for weight loss, muscle gain, or maintaining your current weight? Do you have any dietary restrictions or allergies to accommodate? Tailoring your meal plan to your specific needs ensures that you stay on track and enjoy your meals along the way.

The Benefits of Batch Cooking

Batch cooking is a meal prepping technique that involves making larger quantities of food than you need for a single meal and then storing the extra portions for later use. This approach is a time-saving game-changer. Instead of cooking every meal from scratch, you can prepare several servings at once, reducing your time in the kitchen during the week. Batch cooking is particularly beneficial for dishes that freeze well, such as soups, stews, casseroles, and grains like rice and quinoa. You can prepare a large batch, portion it into individual containers, and freeze them. When you're ready to eat, simply heat and enjoy. This is a fantastic option for those evenings when you're too tired or busy to cook. Additionally, batch cooking allows you to take advantage of sales and discounts at the grocery store. When you find a great deal on chicken, beef, or your favorite vegetables, you can buy them in bulk and use batch cooking to prepare and store meals for the future. This not only saves you money but also ensures that you always have a variety of ingredients at your fingertips.

Smart Grocery Shopping for Meal Prepping
A successful meal prep journey begins with a well-thought-out grocery list. Before you hit the supermarket, take some time to plan your shopping trip. Start by reviewing your meal plan and identifying the ingredients you'll need for the week. Make a list, and stick to it as closely as possible to avoid impulse purchases. When shopping for meal prep, focus on purchasing whole, minimally processed foods. Fresh fruits and vegetables, lean proteins, whole grains, and healthy fats should make up the bulk of your grocery cart. These whole foods are nutrient-dense and provide the essential vitamins, minerals, and fiber your body needs to thrive. Consider the layout of your local grocery store when making your list. Begin with the produce section, where you can stock up on fresh fruits and vegetables. Move on to the meat or plant-based protein section to select your protein sources. Next, head to the grains and legumes aisle for items like rice, quinoa, and beans. Don't forget the dairy or dairy alternatives section for yogurt, milk, or plant-based alternatives. When shopping for perishable items like fruits and vegetables, choose those that are in-season and on sale to save money. You can also buy frozen fruits and vegetables, which retain their nutrients and are often more budget-friendly. For proteins, consider buying in bulk and freezing what you won't use immediately.

Efficient Meal Prep Techniques
Now that you have your meal plan and groceries ready, it's time to roll up your sleeves and start meal prepping. Here are some efficient techniques and tips to make the process smoother:
1. Set aside dedicated time: Choose a specific day and time each week for your meal prep session. Consistency is key, so make it a non-negotiable part of your routine.

2. Organize your workspace: Before you begin cooking, make sure your kitchen is clean and organized. Gather all the necessary equipment and containers, so you don't waste time searching for items later.

3. Multi-task: While one dish is simmering on the stove, you can chop vegetables or prepare another part of your meal. Utilize your time efficiently by working on multiple components simultaneously.

4. Use time-saving appliances: Invest in kitchen appliances like a slow cooker, instant pot, or food processor to expedite cooking tasks. These tools can help you prepare meals with minimal effort.

5. Portion mindfully: When dividing your meals into portions, consider your dietary goals and caloric needs. Use kitchen scales or measuring cups to ensure accuracy.

6. Label and date: Properly label your meal containers with the date of preparation and any necessary reheating instructions. This helps you keep track of freshness and prevents food waste.

Overcoming Common Challenges

While meal prepping offers numerous benefits, it's not without its challenges. Let's address some common hurdles you might encounter and how to overcome them.

1. Time Constraints: Many people believe that meal prepping takes too much time. While it does require an initial investment of time, the long-term time savings and health benefits make it worthwhile. Start small, perhaps with one meal a day, and gradually increase your meal prep efforts as you become more comfortable with the process.

2. Lack of Variety: Some individuals worry that meal prepping will lead to monotonous, repetitive meals. Combat this by experimenting with different recipes and cuisines. Explore new ingredients and flavor combinations to keep your meals exciting and enjoyable.

3. Food Storage and Spoilage: Proper food storage is essential to prevent spoilage and maintain freshness. Invest in a variety of meal containers, both reusable and disposable, to accommodate different meal sizes and types. Educate yourself on the proper storage methods for different foods to maximize shelf life.

4. Travel and Social Events: Meal prepping doesn't mean you can't enjoy dining out or attending social gatherings. Plan ahead for such

occasions by preparing a meal or snack to take with you. When dining out, opt for healthier menu choices and practice portion control.

5. Burnout: Some people may experience meal prep burnout if they feel overwhelmed by the process. Prevent burnout by keeping your meal prep sessions enjoyable. Listen to your favorite music or podcast while cooking, involve family members in the process, or make it a social activity by prepping with friends.

The Long-Term Benefits of Meal Prepping

Meal prepping is not a short-term solution; it's a long-term lifestyle change that can yield a multitude of benefits. Let's explore some of these benefits and how they can positively impact your health and well-being. Meal prepping offers a multitude of benefits, making it a valuable tool for weight management. By planning and preparing your meals, you gain control over portion sizes and can make healthier food choices consistently. This approach empowers you to achieve and maintain a healthy weight by ensuring that your meals are well-balanced and aligned with your dietary goals. Furthermore, meal prepping provides an opportunity to focus on nutrient-dense foods that are rich in essential vitamins, minerals, and fiber. When you take charge of your meal preparation, you can select ingredients that contribute to improved overall nutrition and better health outcomes. This emphasis on nutrient-rich choices can have a profound impact on your well-being over time. Financially, meal prepping can lead to significant savings. Regularly dining out or ordering takeout can quickly deplete your wallet. Meal prepping allows you to make cost-effective choices by purchasing ingredients in bulk and minimizing food waste. By investing a bit of time upfront, you can enjoy substantial financial benefits in the long run. In terms of time efficiency, meal prepping is a game-changer. Over time, it saves you precious hours during the week. With pre-made meals readily available, you can quickly heat and enjoy your dishes, significantly reducing the time spent on cooking and cleaning. This newfound time can be channeled into other activities or simply used for relaxation and self-care. One of the most significant stressors related to daily meal decisions is eliminated through meal prepping. You no longer need to wonder about what to eat or worry about making unhealthy choices when you're hungry and pressed for time. Meal prepping provides a clear plan and removes the uncertainty, allowing you to approach mealtime with confidence and ease. The quality of the food you consume is another aspect that greatly benefits from meal prepping. When you prepare your meals at home, you have full control over the quality of the ingredients you use. You can opt for organic produce, lean proteins, and whole grains, ensuring that your meals are of the highest quality and align with your health and wellness goals. Meal prepping is a customizable approach that caters to your specific dietary needs and preferences. Whether you follow a vegetarian, vegan, gluten-free, or any other specialized diet, meal prep can accommodate your requirements. It empowers you to tailor your meals to your unique tastes and nutritional needs. Over time, meal prepping fosters the development of healthier eating habits. It encourages mindful eating, portion control, and a greater awareness of the nutritional content of your food. These habits become ingrained in your daily routine, leading to lasting improvements in your dietary choices and overall well-being. Perhaps one of the most empowering aspects of meal prepping is the control it gives you over your dietary decisions. You become both the chef and the curator of your meals, making choices that align with your health and wellness goals. This sense of empowerment translates into a more conscious approach to nutrition, where food becomes nourishment, and eating becomes a mindful act. In embracing the meal prepping lifestyle, you may find a profound shift in your relationship with food. Food transcends mere sustenance; it becomes a source of nourishment, health, and empowerment. Eating becomes a conscious and positive act, leading to a more profound and mindful approach to nutrition that enriches your life in countless ways. Incorporating meal prepping into your life is a transformative journey that offers a multitude of benefits for your health, time, and finances. It's a powerful strategy that empowers you to make thoughtful, health-conscious choices and take control of your dietary habits. Meal prepping is not just about convenience; it's about building a healthier, happier you. As you embark on this journey, keep in mind that meal prepping is a flexible and customizable approach.

You can start small and gradually increase your efforts as you become more comfortable with the process. Experiment with different recipes, ingredients, and cuisines to keep your meals exciting and enjoyable. Remember that the goal is not perfection but progress. Embrace the occasional setbacks or challenges as opportunities to learn and grow. Whether your aim is weight loss, improved nutrition, or simply a more organized and stress-free approach to mealtime, meal prepping can be your ally in achieving those goals. So, take that first step into the world of meal prepping, and unlock the potential for a healthier, happier, and more empowered you. Your culinary adventure awaits, and the rewards are both immediate and enduring. Happy meal prepping!

Essential Kitchen Tools and Supplies

The kitchen is the heart of the home, where culinary magic happens and delicious meals are created. To cook efficiently and with finesse, it's essential to have the right tools and supplies at your disposal. In this comprehensive guide, we will explore the must-have kitchen equipment and supplies that every home chef, from novice to experienced, should consider. Whether you're looking to upgrade your kitchen or just starting your culinary journey, understanding the importance of these essential items can elevate your cooking experience and inspire your inner chef.

Knives: The Backbone of Your Kitchen
Knives are the backbone of any kitchen, and having a set of quality knives is non-negotiable. A well-maintained knife can make slicing, dicing, chopping, and mincing a breeze. Here are the types of knives every kitchen should have:
1. Chef's Knife: This versatile, all-purpose knife is the workhorse of the kitchen. It's ideal for a wide range of tasks, from slicing vegetables to chopping herbs and even carving meat. Invest in a high-quality chef's knife that feels comfortable in your hand.
2. Paring Knife: A small, sharp paring knife is perfect for delicate tasks like peeling fruits, deveining shrimp, or creating intricate garnishes. It offers precision and control when working with smaller ingredients.
3. Serrated Bread Knife: The serrated edge of a bread knife is designed to slice through bread without crushing it. It's also handy

for cutting through tomatoes and other foods with a tough exterior and a soft interior.

4. Utility Knife: A utility knife is a mid-sized knife that falls between a chef's knife and a paring knife in terms of versatility. It's great for tasks that require a little more finesse than a chef's knife can provide.

5. Santoku Knife: This Japanese-style knife is known for its exceptional slicing and dicing capabilities. It's a fantastic alternative to a chef's knife and is well-suited for precision cutting.

To maintain your knives' sharpness, invest in a honing rod and learn how to use it properly. Regularly sharpening your knives is essential for safe and efficient cutting.

Cutting Boards: A Stable Surface

A sturdy cutting board is essential for preparing ingredients safely and effectively. Here are the most common types:

1. Wooden Cutting Boards: Wooden boards are gentle on knife edges and have natural antibacterial properties. They require regular maintenance, including oiling and seasoning, to prevent cracking and warping.

2. Plastic Cutting Boards: Plastic boards are easy to clean and come in various colors to help prevent cross-contamination when working with different ingredients. However, they can develop deep knife marks over time, which may harbor bacteria if not properly cleaned.

3. Bamboo Cutting Boards: Bamboo is a sustainable and eco-friendly option that is also gentle on knives. Bamboo boards are durable and resistant to moisture, making them a popular choice among many home chefs.

Consider having multiple cutting boards on hand to prevent cross-contamination. Use one for meats, another for vegetables, and a third for fruits to maintain food safety.

Pots and Pans: The Cooking Essentials

A well-rounded set of pots and pans is crucial for creating a wide variety of dishes. Here are the essentials:

1. Saucepan: This versatile pan is perfect for making sauces, soups, and simmering liquids. Look for one with a heavy bottom to prevent scorching.

2. Skillet or Frying Pan: A good-quality skillet is essential for sautéing, frying, searing, and making omelets. Non-stick and stainless steel options are popular choices.

3. Stockpot: For making large batches of soup, chili, or pasta, a stockpot with a roomy capacity is a must-have.

4. Dutch Oven: Dutch ovens are excellent for slow-cooking dishes like stews and braised meats. They can go from the stovetop to the oven, making them incredibly versatile.

5. Baking Sheets and Roasting Pans: Baking sheets are ideal for roasting vegetables, baking cookies, and making sheet pan meals. Roasting pans are designed for larger roasts and poultry.

6. Non-Stick Pan: A non-stick skillet or pan is essential for cooking delicate foods like eggs and fish without them sticking to the surface.

7. Cast Iron Skillet: Cast iron skillets are known for their even heat distribution and exceptional heat retention. They're perfect for searing, frying, and baking.

When choosing pots and pans, prioritize quality over quantity. Invest in durable, heat-responsive cookware that will last for years with proper care. Additionally, consider the type of stovetop you have (induction, gas, electric) to ensure compatibility.

Cooking Utensils: Tools of the Trade

A well-equipped kitchen needs the right cooking utensils to turn raw ingredients into delicious dishes. Here are some essential utensils you'll want to have:

1. Spatula: Spatulas come in various forms, including turners, slotted, and solid. They are versatile tools for flipping, stirring, and serving.

2. Tongs: Tongs are indispensable for gripping and flipping food items, whether it's flipping a steak on the grill or tossing a salad.

3. Whisk: Whisks are used for blending, beating, and emulsifying ingredients. They come in different shapes and sizes, each suited for specific tasks.

4. Ladle: A ladle is essential for serving soups, stews, and sauces. Look for one with a deep bowl and a long handle.

5. Slotted Spoon: This spoon with slots or holes is handy for lifting solids from liquids, such as when serving pasta or draining vegetables.

6. Wooden Spoons: Wooden spoons are gentle on cookware and can be used for stirring, mixing, and sautéing.

7. Measuring Cups and Spoons: Accurate measurements are crucial in cooking and baking. Invest in both dry and liquid measuring cups and a set of measuring spoons.

8. Kitchen Shears: Kitchen shears are versatile tools for cutting herbs, trimming meat, and opening packaging.

9. Microplane Grater/Zester: A microplane grater is perfect for zesting citrus, grating cheese, and adding fine texture to dishes.

10. Colander or Strainer: A colander is essential for draining pasta, rinsing vegetables, and washing fruits.

11. Basting Brush: A basting brush is used for applying marinades, sauces, or melted butter to food items.

12. Pasta Fork: This fork with long, slender tines is designed to twirl and serve pasta effectively.

13. Silicone Spatula: Silicone spatulas are heat-resistant and perfect for scraping every last bit of batter or sauce from bowls and pans.

14. Kitchen Timer: A reliable kitchen timer is essential for precise cooking and baking.

15. Corkscrew and Bottle Opener: If you enjoy wine or bottled beverages, having a corkscrew and bottle opener in your kitchen is practical.

Having the right cooking utensils not only makes cooking easier but also ensures that your food turns out well-prepared and delicious.

Bakeware: Creating Sweet and Savory Delights

For baking enthusiasts and anyone who enjoys whipping up sweet or savory treats, having the right bakeware is essential. Here are the basics:

1. Mixing Bowls: A set of mixing bowls in various sizes is indispensable for combining ingredients, mixing batters, and tossing salads.

2. Baking Pans: Baking pans come in various shapes and sizes, including cake pans, muffin tins, and pie dishes. Make sure you have the essentials for your favorite baked goods.

3. Cookie Sheets: Cookie sheets are perfect for baking cookies, but they can also be used for roasting vegetables or reheating leftovers.

4. Rolling Pin: A rolling pin is a must for rolling out dough for pies, cookies, and pastries.

5. Cooling Racks: Cooling racks allow baked goods to cool evenly by allowing air circulation. They're essential for preventing items like cookies from becoming soggy.

6. Cake Stand and Decorating Tools: If you enjoy baking cakes and decorating them, a cake stand and decorating tools like piping bags and tips are a valuable addition to your kitchen.

Small Appliances: Enhancing Efficiency

Small kitchen appliances can enhance your cooking and baking efficiency. Consider adding these to your collection:

1. Food Processor: A food processor can chop, slice, dice, and puree ingredients quickly. It's excellent for making sauces, dressings, and dips.

2. Blender: Blenders are versatile tools for making smoothies, soups, sauces, and purees. High-speed blenders can even pulverize nuts and grains.

3. Stand Mixer: Stand mixers are a baking enthusiast's best friend. They make tasks like whipping egg whites, kneading dough, and mixing batters effortless.

4. Hand Mixer: For those who don't have the space or budget for a stand mixer, a hand mixer is a handy alternative for mixing and beating.

5. Coffee Maker or Electric Kettle: If you're a coffee or tea lover, having a coffee maker or electric kettle can streamline your morning routine.

6. Toaster or Toaster Oven: Toasters are perfect for quickly toasting bread, while toaster ovens can handle a wider variety of tasks, including reheating and broiling.

7. Slow Cooker or Instant Pot: These multi-functional appliances are ideal for slow-cooking soups, stews, and roasts. Instant Pots can also serve as pressure cookers, making them versatile additions to your kitchen.

8. Microwave: While not technically a small appliance, a microwave is a kitchen staple for quickly reheating and defrosting.

Storage Containers: Keeping Food Fresh

Proper food storage is essential for preserving freshness and preventing food waste. Consider these storage options:

1. Food Storage Containers: Invest in a variety of food storage containers, including airtight containers for dry goods, glass containers for leftovers, and plastic containers for meal prep.
2. Freezer Bags: Freezer bags are essential for portioning and freezing soups, sauces, and individual servings of food.
3. Mason Jars: Mason jars are versatile for storing homemade jams, pickles, dressings, and even salads.
4. Aluminum Foil and Plastic Wrap: These kitchen essentials are handy for covering leftovers or wrapping items for the freezer.
5. Reusable Food Wraps: Eco-friendly alternatives like beeswax wraps are perfect for covering bowls and wrapping sandwiches.

Kitchen Gadgets: Simplifying Tasks

There are a plethora of kitchen gadgets and tools that can simplify specific tasks. While not essential, they can make cooking more enjoyable and efficient. Some popular gadgets include garlic presses, citrus juicers, egg separators, and avocado slicers. Consider your cooking habits and which gadgets align with your culinary preferences. Investing in high-quality bakeware and cookware is a smart decision, but it's equally important to ensure their longevity through proper care and maintenance. Here are some valuable tips to keep your kitchen equipment in optimal condition:

Consider handwashing your bakeware and cookware whenever possible. While many kitchen items are labeled as dishwasher safe, handwashing is a gentler approach that helps prevent the degradation of non-stick coatings and preserves the integrity of materials like wood and cast iron. When cooking with non-stick pans, be mindful of the utensils you use. Avoid using metal utensils that can scratch the surface. Instead, opt for utensils made of silicone, wood, or plastic to protect the non-stick coating and maintain the cookware's performance. For cast iron skillets, regular seasoning is essential to preserve their non-stick surface and prevent rust. Seasoning involves applying a thin layer of oil and heating the skillet to create a protective coating that enhances its longevity. Proper knife storage is crucial for both safety and blade maintenance. Invest in a knife block, magnetic strip, or blade guards to protect your knives, prevent injury, and keep the blades sharp. Regularly inspect your cookware and bakeware for signs of wear and tear. Look out for peeling non-stick coatings, warped pans, or loose handles. Items that show signs of deterioration should be replaced promptly to ensure safe and efficient cooking. Certain types of cookware may require specific cleaning tools for optimal care. For example, stainless steel pans may benefit from the use of a stainless steel cleaner to maintain their shine and prevent discoloration. Always adhere to the manufacturer's instructions for care and maintenance. Different materials, such as stainless steel, cast iron, and non-stick coatings, may have unique requirements to ensure their longevity and performance. Incorporating these tips into your kitchen routine will help you preserve the quality and durability of your bakeware and cookware. By taking the time to care for these essential kitchen tools, you'll continue to enjoy their benefits in your culinary endeavors for years to come. Having the right kitchen tools and supplies is essential for every home chef. Whether you're a seasoned cook or just starting, a well-equipped kitchen allows you to explore your culinary creativity, experiment with new recipes, and cook with confidence. Investing in high-quality knives, pots and pans, cooking utensils, bakeware, and small appliances can make your kitchen experience more enjoyable and efficient. Remember that quality and durability should guide your choices when building your kitchen arsenal. Take the time to properly care for and maintain your kitchen equipment to ensure it serves you well for years to come. With the right tools at your disposal, you can craft culinary delights that will delight your taste buds and those of your loved ones. So, step into your kitchen, armed with the essentials, and let your culinary journey begin. Happy cooking!

Planning Your Meals and Budget

Meal planning and budgeting are essential life skills that can help you improve your eating habits and manage your finances more effectively. By combining the art of meal planning with smart budgeting strategies, you can achieve your health and financial goals simultaneously. Let's explore the benefits of meal planning, how to get started, and how it intersects with budgeting.

The Benefits of Meal Planning

Meal planning offers a range of benefits that can positively impact your life. One of the most significant advantages is that it promotes healthier eating habits. When you plan your meals in advance, you have the opportunity to make intentional and nutritious food choices. This means incorporating a variety of food groups into your diet, including fruits, vegetables, lean proteins, whole grains, and healthy fats. By designing your meals, you're more likely to avoid impulse decisions that lead to unhealthy eating. Another advantage of meal planning is better portion control. You can pre-determine serving sizes and avoid overeating, which is especially helpful if you're aiming for weight management or other dietary goals. Furthermore, meal planning reduces food waste by helping you purchase only what you need. No more forgotten ingredients languishing in the back of your fridge, which not only saves money but is also environmentally friendly. Time efficiency is another significant benefit. Planning your meals means you know exactly what to cook each day, eliminating the need to make rushed decisions when you're hungry and tired. This can save you precious minutes during busy weekdays. Plus, it can lead to cost savings by reducing the temptation to order takeout or dine out when you have pre-planned meals ready at home. Variety and exploration are encouraged by meal planning. It pushes you to try new recipes and cuisines, preventing culinary boredom. Experimenting with different dishes keeps your meals exciting and enjoyable, making healthy eating a sustainable lifestyle. Lastly, meal planning reduces the stress associated with mealtime decisions. You won't find yourself scrambling to figure out what to cook or eat when you're already famished. Knowing what's on the menu in advance eliminates mealtime stress, making your overall dining experience more pleasant.

Getting Started with Meal Planning
Meal planning doesn't have to be complicated. Here's a simplified guide to help you start your journey:
Begin by setting clear meal planning goals. Are you looking to eat healthier, lose weight, save time, or all of the above? Your goals will guide your meal planning decisions. Create a meal calendar or schedule. Designate a specific time each week to plan your meals. Whether you prefer a digital calendar or a physical planner, having a designated space for meal planning can keep you organized. Before you start planning, take stock of what you already have in your kitchen. This prevents duplicate purchases and ensures you

use up ingredients that are close to their expiration dates. Choose recipes that align with your goals and dietary preferences. Consider dishes that are well-balanced and include a variety of foods. Gradually expand your meal planning from one meal a day to others as you become more comfortable with the process.

Create a detailed shopping list based on your chosen recipes. Organize the list by food category to make your grocery shopping more efficient. Be specific about quantities to avoid overbuying.

After your grocery trip, set aside time for ingredient preparation. Wash, chop, and portion vegetables, proteins, and grains to streamline meal preparation during the week. Store prepped ingredients and meals in an organized manner. Use containers that are easy to access and label them with preparation dates and any reheating instructions. Periodically review your meal plan and adjust it as needed to accommodate changing preferences or dietary needs. Remember to stay flexible, as life can be unpredictable, and it's okay to deviate from your plan occasionally. Be patient and open to refining your approach as you gain more experience with meal planning.

Budgeting and Meal Planning: A Winning Combination
Meal planning and budgeting work in harmony to help you achieve your financial goals while enjoying nutritious and delicious meals. Here's how they intersect:

Begin by establishing a food budget that aligns with your financial goals. Consider factors such as your income, household size, and spending priorities. Your food budget should cover both groceries and dining out. Keep a close eye on your food-related expenses by tracking receipts and transactions. Categorize your spending to understand where your money is going, which will help you identify areas where you can cut costs. Allocate a portion of your food budget to each meal, such as breakfast, lunch, and dinner. Adjust these allocations based on your financial goals and dietary needs. When planning your meals, be mindful of your meal budget allocations. Choose recipes and ingredients that fit within your budget constraints. Look for cost-effective options like buying in bulk or using leftovers creatively. Stick to your shopping list and avoid impulse purchases. Compare prices, consider store brands or generic options, and take advantage of sales and discounts to maximize savings. Incorporate budget-friendly staples like rice, pasta, beans, and root vegetables into your meals. These ingredients are versatile and can form the basis of many dishes. Plan meals that yield leftovers, which can be repurposed into new dishes. For example, a roasted chicken can become chicken salad or chicken soup the next day. Consider reducing the frequency of dining out and allocate those funds to your grocery budget. When you do dine out, choose budget-friendly options like lunch specials or happy hour deals. Prevent food waste to save money and reduce environmental impact. Use leftover ingredients creatively, freeze items for future use, and practice proper food storage to extend shelf life. Regularly review your food budget and meal plan to ensure they align with your financial goals. Make adjustments as needed to stay on track. Meal planning and budgeting are valuable skills that can transform your eating habits and financial management. By proactively planning your meals, you can make healthier food choices, reduce food waste, save time, and enjoy cost savings. Combining meal planning with effective budgeting strategies allows you to align your nutrition goals with your financial objectives. Remember that both meal planning and budgeting are flexible approaches that can be tailored to your unique goals and preferences. As you embark on this journey, be patient with yourself and open to making adjustments as needed. Over time, you'll develop a meal planning and budgeting routine that seamlessly fits into your lifestyle, leading to greater financial freedom and a healthier relationship with food. So, start planning your meals with intention, and watch as it not only transforms your plate but also your financial well-being.

Grocery Shopping Tips for Weight Loss

Grocery shopping plays a pivotal role in your weight loss journey. The choices you make at the grocery store can significantly impact your ability to achieve and maintain a healthy weight. By adopting smart shopping strategies and making mindful decisions, you can stock your kitchen with nutritious foods that support your weight loss goals. In this guide, we will explore essential grocery shopping tips tailored to weight loss, helping you make informed choices and build a foundation for a healthier lifestyle.

The Importance of Smart Grocery Shopping

Before diving into specific tips, let's underscore the importance of smart grocery shopping in your weight loss journey. The supermarket is where your food choices take shape, and it's the place where you have the most control over what you consume. When you shop strategically, you set yourself up for success by:

1. Nourishing Your Body: Smart shopping allows you to fill your cart with nutrient-dense foods that provide essential vitamins, minerals, and fiber. These foods support your overall health and help you feel full and satisfied.

2. Controlling Portions: By choosing appropriate portion sizes and avoiding tempting high-calorie snacks, you can manage your calorie intake more effectively. Portion control is a key element of weight loss.

3. Minimizing Temptation: Grocery stores are filled with tempting but unhealthy foods. Smart shopping involves avoiding or limiting these temptations, making it easier to stick to your weight loss plan.

4. Saving Money: Shopping with a plan reduces impulse purchases and wasteful spending. It can help you stay within your budget while prioritizing healthier options.

5. Enhancing Meal Planning: The ingredients you bring home from the grocery store are the building blocks of your meals. Smart shopping complements meal planning and encourages you to prepare balanced, weight-loss-friendly dishes.

Now, let's delve into practical grocery shopping tips to help you make the most of your trips to the store.

Tip 1: Plan Your Shopping List

One of the most effective strategies for smart grocery shopping is to plan your list in advance. Take some time to outline your meals and snacks for the week. Having a clear plan helps you:

- Avoid Impulse Buys: With a list in hand, you're less likely to veer off course and make impulsive, unhealthy purchases.

- Stay Focused: You'll be more efficient in the store, reducing the chances of wandering into tempting aisles filled with processed snacks and sugary treats.

- Minimize Food Waste: Planning your meals ensures you buy only what you need, reducing the likelihood of perishable items going to waste.

When creating your shopping list, include a variety of foods from different food groups. Prioritize fruits, vegetables, lean proteins, whole grains, and healthy fats. These foods are essential for a balanced, weight-loss-friendly diet.

Tip 2: Shop the Perimeter

Navigating the layout of the grocery store strategically can make a significant difference in your shopping choices. Typically, the perimeter of the store is where you'll find fresh, whole foods like produce, lean meats, dairy, and seafood. These are the items you should focus on during your shopping trip. The interior aisles, on the other hand, often contain highly processed, calorie-dense products. While there may be some healthy options within the aisles (such as whole-grain pasta or canned beans), it's important to approach these areas with caution. When you venture into the inner aisles, stick to your list and avoid getting sidetracked by tempting, less nutritious options.

Tip 3: Read Nutrition Labels

Nutrition labels are your best friend when it comes to making informed food choices. They provide valuable information about serving sizes, calorie counts, and nutrient content. Here's what to look for on nutrition labels:

- Serving Size: Pay attention to serving sizes to ensure you're consuming an appropriate portion. Sometimes a package may contain multiple servings.
- Calories per Serving: Check the calorie count per serving to gauge the energy content of the food.
- Macronutrients: Look at the amounts of protein, carbohydrates, and fat. Focus on foods that are higher in protein and fiber and lower in added sugars and saturated fats.
- Ingredients: Review the ingredient list for any added sugars, unhealthy fats (like trans fats), and artificial additives. Opt for foods with simple, recognizable ingredients.
- Nutrient Percentages: Some labels provide the percentage of daily recommended intake for certain nutrients. Use this information to make choices that align with your dietary goals.

Nutrition labels empower you to compare products and select the healthiest options. Be particularly cautious of items with hidden sugars and excessive salt content.

Tip 4: Buy Fresh and Frozen Produce
Fruits and vegetables are essential components of a weight-loss-friendly diet, but they can be a challenge to keep fresh throughout the week. To ensure you always have access to produce, consider buying a combination of fresh and frozen options. Fresh produce is fantastic for its variety and flavor, but it can spoil quickly. Plan to use fresh items earlier in the week and save frozen options for later. Frozen fruits and vegetables are typically flash-frozen at their peak ripeness, preserving their nutritional value. They're convenient, have a longer shelf life, and can be a lifesaver when you're running low on fresh produce.

Tip 5: Beware of Hidden Sugars and Sodium
Many packaged and processed foods contain hidden sugars and excessive sodium, which can thwart your weight loss efforts. Sugar and salt can be added to a wide range of products, from salad dressings to canned soups. To make informed choices:
- Check Ingredient Lists: Look for added sugars and sodium in the ingredient list. These may appear as various names, including sucrose, high fructose corn syrup, and sodium chloride.
- Compare Products: Compare similar products and choose the one with lower sugar and sodium content. Opt for products labeled "no added sugar" or "low sodium" when available.
- Be Mindful of Sauces and Condiments: Be cautious with condiments like ketchup, barbecue sauce, and salad dressings, as they can be high in added sugars and sodium. Consider making your own healthier versions at home.

Tip 6: Choose Lean Proteins
Protein is a crucial component of a weight-loss-friendly diet. It helps you feel full and satisfied, preventing overeating. When shopping for protein sources, prioritize lean options such as skinless poultry, lean cuts of beef or pork, fish, tofu, tempeh, legumes (beans, lentils, chickpeas), and low-fat dairy products. Limit your consumption of processed meats like bacon, sausages, and deli meats, as they are often high in saturated fats and sodium. Instead, choose fresh, whole protein sources and incorporate them into your meals for a balanced diet.

Tip 7: Practice Mindful Snacking
Snacking can either support your weight loss goals or hinder them, depending on your choices. When selecting snacks, opt for options that are nutrient-dense and satisfying. Consider these tips:
- Portion Control: Choose snacks that come in portion-controlled packaging or pre-portion them at home to avoid overeating.
- Balanced Snacks: Pair a source of protein (e.g., yogurt, nuts, or hummus) with a serving of fruits or vegetables for a balanced, filling snack.
- Minimize Processed Snacks: Highly processed snacks like chips and sugary cereals
 should be enjoyed sparingly. Instead, reach for whole-food options like air-popped popcorn or whole-grain crackers.
- Hydration: Sometimes, thirst is mistaken for hunger. Stay hydrated by drinking water throughout the day, which can help reduce unnecessary snacking.

Tip 8: Shop with a Full Stomach
Grocery shopping on an empty stomach can be a recipe for disaster. When you're hungry, you're more likely to make impulsive decisions and grab unhealthy snacks that satisfy immediate cravings. To avoid this, plan your shopping trips after you've had a meal or a substantial snack. Shopping on a full stomach can help you stay focused on your shopping list and make healthier choices.

Tip 9: Avoid Sugary Beverages
Calories from sugary beverages can quickly add up and derail your weight loss efforts. When you shop, steer clear of sodas, sweetened fruit juices, energy drinks, and other high-calorie drinks. Instead, opt for healthier alternatives like water, herbal tea, unsweetened iced tea, or sparkling water with a splash of citrus.

Tip 10: Don't Be Afraid to Explore
While it's essential to stick to your shopping list and make mindful choices, don't be afraid to explore new foods and ingredients. Trying new recipes and incorporating unfamiliar foods into your diet can keep your meals exciting and prevent monotony, which can lead to overindulgence in less healthy options.

Empowering Your Weight Loss Journey through Smart Shopping

Grocery shopping is a fundamental aspect of your weight loss journey, and it's a place where you have the power to make positive choices. By planning your shopping list, focusing on nutrient-dense options, reading nutrition labels, and avoiding hidden sugars and sodium, you can stock your kitchen with foods that support your weight loss goals. Remember to prioritize fresh and frozen produce, choose lean proteins, and practice mindful snacking. These strategies, combined with healthy cooking and portion control, can set you on a path to successful and sustainable weight loss. Embrace the process of smart grocery shopping as an opportunity to nourish your body, make conscious decisions, and build a foundation for a healthier lifestyle. Over time, these habits will become second nature, empowering you to make confident choices that align with your weight loss goals. So, step into the supermarket with knowledge and intention, and watch as your cart fills with the ingredients for a healthier, happier you. Your weight loss journey starts with every thoughtful choice you make at the grocery store.

Chapter 2
Weekly Meal Prep Calendar

Week 1: Embarking on Your Weight Loss Journey

Welcome to Week 1 of your weight loss journey! This is the beginning of a transformative process that will help you achieve your health and wellness goals. In this crucial first week, we will lay the foundation for success by focusing on essential aspects of weight loss, including setting clear goals, understanding your current habits, and making mindful choices. Let's embark on this journey together and take the first steps toward a healthier you.

Day 1: Setting Clear Goals
Today is all about defining your weight loss goals. To succeed, you need a clear and compelling reason to embark on this journey. Take some time to reflect on why you want to lose weight. Is it to improve your health, boost your confidence, or increase your energy levels? Write down your goals, making sure they are specific, measurable, achievable, relevant, and time-bound (SMART goals). Having a clear vision of what you want to achieve will keep you motivated throughout this journey.

Day 2: Assessing Your Current Habits
Understanding your current habits is a crucial step in your weight loss journey. Take an honest look at your eating, exercise, and lifestyle habits. Keep a food diary for the day, recording everything you eat and drink. Pay attention to portion sizes, meal timing, and any emotional triggers that lead to overeating. Also, assess your physical activity level and daily routines. This self-awareness will help you identify areas for improvement.

Day 3: Creating a Balanced Meal Plan
Today, we'll begin building a balanced meal plan. Start by calculating your daily calorie needs based on your goals and activity level. You can use online tools or consult with a healthcare

professional for guidance. Next, plan your meals for the week, ensuring they include a variety of nutrient-dense foods like fruits, vegetables, lean proteins, whole grains, and healthy fats. Portion control is key, so be mindful of serving sizes. Aim for balanced meals that provide sustained energy and keep you feeling full.

Day 4: Stocking a Healthy Kitchen

Your kitchen plays a central role in your weight loss journey. Today, take the time to clean out your pantry, refrigerator, and freezer. Remove any tempting, unhealthy foods that could derail your progress. Replace them with nutritious alternatives, such as fresh produce, lean proteins, and whole grains. Having a well-stocked, healthy kitchen makes it easier to make mindful choices and prepare balanced meals.

Day 5: Starting an Exercise Routine

Exercise is a crucial component of weight loss and overall health. Begin your exercise routine with a focus on activities you enjoy. Whether it's walking, cycling, dancing, or yoga, find an activity that makes you feel good. Start with a manageable time commitment, aiming for at least 30 minutes of moderate-intensity exercise most days of the week. Gradually increase the duration and intensity as you build strength and stamina.

Day 6: Mindful Eating Practices

Today, we'll delve into mindful eating practices. Mindful eating involves paying full attention to your food and eating with intention. Practice eating without distractions, such as phones or TV. Take your time to savor each bite, noticing the flavors, textures, and sensations. Listen to your body's hunger and fullness cues, eating until you're satisfied, not stuffed. Mindful eating helps prevent overeating and fosters a healthier relationship with food.

Day 7: Seeking Support and Accountability

Support and accountability are essential on your weight loss journey. Today, reach out to friends, family members, or a support group who can encourage and motivate you. Share your goals and progress with them. Additionally, consider seeking professional support from a registered dietitian, personal trainer, or therapist, depending on your needs. Having a support system in place will help you stay on track and overcome challenges.

A Strong Start to Your Journey
Congratulations on completing Week 1 of your weight loss journey! By setting clear goals, assessing your habits, creating a balanced meal plan, stocking a healthy kitchen, starting an exercise routine, practicing mindful eating, and seeking support, you've taken significant steps toward a healthier you. Remember that this is just the beginning, and the path ahead may have its challenges. Stay committed, stay positive, and keep your goals in sight. You have the power to transform your life and achieve lasting weight loss success. Week 2 awaits, where we'll dive deeper into nutrition, exercise, and habit-building strategies. Keep moving forward on this empowering journey to better health and well-being!

Week 2: Navigating Nutrition and Fitness

Welcome to Week 2 of your weight loss journey! By now, you've laid a strong foundation by setting clear goals, assessing your habits, and creating a balanced meal plan. In this second week, we will delve deeper into the essential aspects of nutrition and fitness to help you make informed choices and develop a sustainable routine. Let's continue on this path towards a healthier and more vibrant you.

Day 1: Understanding Macronutrients
To make informed choices about your diet, it's crucial to understand macronutrients—carbohydrates, proteins, and fats. Each macronutrient plays a unique role in your body:
- Carbohydrates: They are your body's primary source of energy. Focus on complex carbohydrates like whole grains, fruits, and vegetables, which provide sustained energy and fiber.
- Proteins: Essential for muscle repair and overall health. Include lean sources like poultry, fish, beans, and tofu in your meals.
- Fats: Healthy fats, like those found in avocados, nuts, and olive oil, support brain function and nutrient absorption. Limit saturated and trans fats found in fried and processed foods.
Today, examine your meal plan to ensure it includes a balance of these macronutrients to meet your nutritional needs.

Day 2: Portion Control and Mindful Eating
Portion control is a fundamental aspect of weight loss. Even healthy foods can contribute to weight gain if consumed in excessive amounts. Practice portion control by:
- Using smaller plates and utensils to trick your brain into thinking you're eating more.
- Measuring and weighing your food to become more aware of portion sizes.
- Serving yourself in the kitchen, rather than at the table, to avoid second helpings.
Additionally, continue to practice mindful eating by savoring each bite, listening to your body's hunger cues, and eating without distractions.

Day 3: Building Healthy Habits
Developing healthy habits is key to long-term success. Start by setting a specific habit-related goal, such as drinking more water, eating more vegetables, or getting enough sleep. Break this goal down into smaller, manageable steps. For example, if your goal is to drink more water, you can start by drinking a glass before each meal. Over time, these small changes will become ingrained habits that support your weight loss journey.

Day 4: Hydration and Weight Loss
Staying hydrated is essential for overall health and can aid in weight loss. Water helps control appetite, supports metabolism, and improves digestion. Aim to drink at least 8 glasses (64 ounces) of water a day. To make hydration more appealing, try infused water with slices of citrus, cucumber, or herbs. Additionally, reduce or eliminate sugary drinks like soda, which can contribute to excess calorie intake.

Day 5: The Role of Fiber
Dietary fiber is a weight loss ally. It keeps you feeling full and satisfied, preventing overeating. It also supports digestive health and helps control blood sugar levels. Increase your fiber intake by incorporating more fruits, vegetables, whole grains, and legumes into your meals. Aim for at least 25 grams of fiber per day.

Day 6: Effective Meal Prepping

Meal prepping can streamline your week and make healthy eating more convenient. Set aside time each week to plan and prepare meals in advance. Consider batch-cooking grains, proteins, and vegetables, and store them in individual containers. This practice ensures you always have nutritious options on hand, reducing the temptation to make unhealthy choices when you're short on time.

Day 7: Introduction to Exercise

Physical activity is a vital component of weight loss and overall health. If you haven't already, it's time to incorporate regular exercise into your routine. Start with activities you enjoy, whether it's walking, swimming, or dancing. The goal is to gradually increase your activity level over time. Aim for at least 150 minutes of moderate-intensity aerobic activity per week, as recommended by health experts.

Building a Solid Foundation

Congratulations on completing Week 2 of your weight loss journey! You've expanded your knowledge of macronutrients, practiced portion control, and deepened your understanding of healthy habits. As you continue your journey, remember that consistency and patience are key. Developing lifelong habits takes time, and setbacks may occur along the way. Stay focused on your goals, stay adaptable, and keep moving forward. Week 3 will bring further insights into nutrition, exercise, and mindset strategies to help you on your path to sustainable weight loss. Remember that this journey is about more than just shedding pounds—it's about embracing a healthier, happier lifestyle. Keep your motivation high, and let your commitment to a healthier you drive your progress. Week 3 awaits with more tools and knowledge to support your transformation.

Week 3: Exploring Nutrient-Rich Options

Welcome to Week 3 of your transformative weight loss journey! By now, you've established a strong foundation by setting goals, assessing your habits, and diving into essential aspects of nutrition and fitness. In this third week, we will continue to deepen your understanding of these key areas while also exploring the importance of mindset and motivation. Let's keep moving forward on this path toward a healthier, happier you.

Day 1: Balanced Eating Patterns

Balanced eating is essential for long-term weight management and overall health. Today, focus on building balanced meals that include:
- Protein: Lean sources like chicken, fish, beans, and tofu provide satiety and support muscle maintenance.
- Fiber: Incorporate plenty of fruits, vegetables, and whole grains to help control hunger and maintain steady blood sugar levels.
- Healthy Fats: Include sources like avocados, nuts, and olive oil to support heart health and nutrient absorption.
- Portion Control: Continue practicing portion control to avoid overeating, even with healthy foods.

Balanced eating is your compass on this journey. It's not about deprivation but about nourishing your body with the right foods. As you continue crafting balanced meals, remember that this approach is sustainable and enjoyable. It's not a quick fix but a lasting solution to a healthier you. Keep experimenting with new recipes and flavors to keep your taste buds excited. Embrace the joy of eating well and feeling good. Remember that variety is key to a balanced diet, so aim to include a diverse range of foods in your meals.

Day 2: Mindful Snacking

Snacking can either support your weight loss goals or derail them, depending on your choices. Today, focus on mindful snacking by:
- Choosing nutrient-dense snacks like yogurt, nuts, or whole fruit.
- Avoiding mindless snacking in front of the TV or computer.
- Listening to your body's hunger cues and eating when you're genuinely hungry, not out of boredom or stress.

Mindful snacking can help you stay on track and prevent overindulgence in less healthy options.

Your journey is about making mindful choices that support your well-being. Today, embrace the art of mindful snacking. By savoring each bite and listening to your body, you're creating a healthier relationship with food. This practice isn't just about what you eat; it's about how you eat. It's a small, daily act of self-care that adds up to significant transformation over time.

Day 3: The Power of Meal Timing
Meal timing can influence your metabolism and energy levels. Aim to eat regular, balanced meals and snacks throughout the day to:
- Maintain steady energy levels and prevent energy crashes.
- Avoid excessive hunger that can lead to overeating.
- Support your metabolism by spreading out your calorie intake.
Experiment with meal timing to find a schedule that works best for your body and lifestyle.
The timing of your meals can be a powerful ally in your weight loss journey. By nourishing your body regularly, you're maintaining steady energy levels and preventing those pesky energy crashes that lead to unhealthy cravings. This is a reminder that you're not just watching the clock; you're investing in your health and well-being with every balanced meal and snack.

Day 4: Strength Training Benefits
Strength training is a valuable addition to your exercise routine. It helps build lean muscle mass, which can boost metabolism and aid in weight loss. Consider incorporating strength training exercises like bodyweight exercises, weight lifting, or resistance bands into your workouts. Aim to include strength training at least two to three times a week.

Day 5: Mindset and Motivation
A positive mindset and strong motivation are crucial for staying on course with your weight loss journey. Reflect on your motivations for wanting to lose weight and remind yourself of these reasons daily. Cultivate a growth mindset by focusing on progress rather than perfection. Be kind to yourself during setbacks, and use them as opportunities to learn and grow.

Day 6: Flexibility in Eating
Today, we'll discuss the importance of flexibility in your eating plan. While structure is essential, it's also essential to allow for flexibility on occasion. Enjoy occasional treats or meals outside your usual plan without guilt. The key is moderation and getting back on track afterward. A flexible approach to eating can make your journey more enjoyable and sustainable.

Day 7: Rest and Recovery

Rest and recovery are often overlooked but critical aspects of any fitness routine. They allow your body to repair and grow stronger. Make sure to include rest days in your exercise schedule to prevent burnout and reduce the risk of injury. Use these days for gentle activities like stretching or leisurely walks to support your overall well-being.

Progress and Persistence

Congratulations on completing Week 3 of your weight loss journey! You've continued to deepen your knowledge of balanced eating, mindful snacking, meal timing, and the benefits of strength training. Additionally, you've explored the importance of mindset, motivation, and flexibility in your approach. These tools and insights will continue to serve you well on your path to sustainable weight loss. As you move forward, remember that progress may not always be linear, and challenges may arise. Stay persistent and focused on your goals, and don't be discouraged by temporary setbacks. Your commitment to a healthier lifestyle is a journey that will lead to lasting change. Embrace each day as an opportunity to learn, grow, and become the healthiest version of yourself. Keep your motivation high, stay resilient, and keep moving toward your goals.

Week 4: Strengthening Your Journey

Congratulations on reaching Week 4 of your incredible weight loss journey! You've already achieved so much, from setting clear goals to deepening your understanding of balanced nutrition, mindful choices, meal timing, and the benefits of strength training. As we delve into this week, we'll continue to explore the essential components of sustainable weight loss, including advanced nutrition strategies, diverse exercise routines, mindfulness techniques, and resilience-building habits. Together, we'll reinforce the strong foundation you've built and empower you to keep moving forward.

Day 1: Advanced Nutrition Strategies

Now that you're well-versed in balanced eating, it's time to explore advanced nutrition strategies. Dive deeper into the world of macronutrients and micronutrients. Pay attention to the quality of your carbohydrates, fats, and proteins. Consider the role of vitamins and minerals in supporting your health. Think of your meals as a canvas, and you're the artist creating a masterpiece of nourishment.

Day 2: Exploring New Fitness Avenues

Variety is the spice of life, and it's also a key factor in maintaining an active lifestyle. Today, venture beyond your comfort zone and explore new fitness avenues. Whether it's trying a new fitness class, hiking a different trail, or experimenting with a different type of exercise equipment, these new experiences not only keep things exciting but also challenge your body in fresh ways.

Day 3: Mindfulness and Stress Reduction

Mindfulness is a powerful tool for managing stress, which can often be a stumbling block on your journey. Spend time today practicing mindfulness techniques like meditation, deep breathing exercises, or yoga. These practices can help you stay centered, reduce emotional eating, and make more conscious choices when faced with stressors.

Day 4: Setting Non-Scale Goals

While the number on the scale is a measure of progress, it's essential not to fixate solely on it. Today, set non-scale goals that celebrate your achievements beyond weight loss. These goals could be related to your fitness level, like running a certain distance or lifting a specific weight. They could also be lifestyle goals, such as fitting into a favorite piece of clothing or having more energy for activities you love.

Day 5: Tracking Progress and Adjusting

Tracking your progress is vital for staying on course. Take some time today to assess how far you've come. Review your goals, and celebrate the milestones you've achieved. If you encounter any challenges or plateaus, don't be discouraged. Instead, consider making adjustments to your meal plan, exercise routine, or mindset strategies. Remember that progress is not always linear, and your journey is about resilience and adaptation.

Day 6: Support and Accountability

Your support system is your strength. Today, reach out to your support network, whether it's friends, family, or fellow journeyers. Share your successes and challenges, and let them be your cheerleaders. Consider finding a workout buddy or an accountability partner to help you stay motivated and on track. Together, you'll navigate this journey with even greater determination.

Day 7: Embracing Rest as Progress

As you reach the end of Week 4, remember that rest is not a pause in your progress but a vital part of it. Today, honor your body by prioritizing rest and recovery. Reflect on how far you've come and appreciate the hard work you've put in. Rest is not a sign of giving up but a demonstration of wisdom and self-care. You're not just transforming your body; you're nurturing your spirit and well-being.

Your Unwavering Commitment

Congratulations on completing Week 4 of your remarkable weight loss journey! You've explored advanced nutrition, diversified your exercise routine, practiced mindfulness, set non-scale goals, and embraced the importance of support and rest. Your commitment to your well-being is unwavering, and your journey is a testament to your resilience. As you move forward into the next phase of your journey, remember that sustainable weight loss is not just about shedding pounds; it's about building a healthier, happier life. Keep the lessons and tools you've gained close to your heart, and let them guide you through the days ahead. You are on a remarkable path of transformation, and your journey is an inspiring example of dedication and self-care. Keep your motivation high, stay adaptable, and keep moving forward. Your commitment to a healthier you is not just a journey—it's a lifelong adventure filled with opportunities for growth and fulfillment.

Chapter 3
Recipes for Weight Loss

Healthy Breakfast Choices: Fueling Your Weight Loss Journey

Breakfast is often hailed as the most important meal of the day, and for a good reason. It sets the tone for your entire day, providing the essential nutrients and energy needed to kickstart your metabolism and keep you satisfied until your next meal. In your weight loss journey, making smart and satisfying breakfast choices is crucial. In this comprehensive guide, we will explore the principles of a healthy breakfast, the benefits it offers for weight loss, and a variety of delicious and nutritious breakfast recipes to keep you on track towards your goals.

The Importance of a Nutrient-Packed Breakfast
A well-balanced breakfast offers a multitude of advantages for individuals embarking on a weight loss journey. Firstly, it jumpstarts your metabolism, effectively revving up your body's calorie-burning engine for the day ahead. This metabolic boost can contribute to more efficient weight management over time. Moreover, a substantial breakfast plays a pivotal role in controlling hunger throughout the day. By satisfying your morning appetite, you're less likely to succumb to overeating or unhealthy snacking later in the day, making it a valuable strategy for weight control. The benefits of breakfast extend beyond weight management, impacting cognitive function as well. A nutritious morning meal enhances concentration, mental clarity, and overall productivity, setting a positive tone for the day ahead. This improved cognitive function can support better decision-making, including choices related to dietary habits. Another crucial aspect of breakfast is its role in stabilizing blood sugar levels. Consuming a balanced breakfast helps regulate blood sugar, reducing the temptation for sugary snacks or erratic eating patterns that can undermine weight loss efforts. Furthermore, breakfast presents an excellent

opportunity to incorporate essential nutrients into your diet. It's a chance to load up on fiber, vitamins, and minerals that contribute to overall health and well-being. These nutrients support various bodily functions and can aid in weight loss by ensuring your body receives the necessary elements for optimal functioning. Breakfast provides the vital energy needed to tackle daily tasks and exercise routines effectively. By fueling your body in the morning, you ensure you have the stamina and vitality required to stay active and make the most of your day, further supporting your weight loss goals. A well-balanced breakfast is a cornerstone of successful weight management. Its ability to boost metabolism, control hunger, enhance cognitive function, stabilize blood sugar, provide essential nutrients, and sustain energy levels makes it an invaluable tool on your weight loss journey. By prioritizing a nutritious breakfast, you set a positive tone for the day and empower yourself to make healthier choices that align with your goals.

Principles of a Healthy Breakfast for Weight Loss

Building a nutritious and weight-loss-friendly breakfast involves following these principles:
1. Balanced Macronutrients: Aim for a combination of carbohydrates, proteins, and healthy fats. This balance helps you stay full and satisfied.
2. Whole Foods: Opt for whole grains, fresh fruits, vegetables, and lean proteins to maximize nutrient intake.
3. Portion Control: Be mindful of portion sizes to avoid overeating.
4. Low Added Sugars: Minimize added sugars in your breakfast choices, as they can lead to energy crashes and cravings later in the day.
5. Hydration: Start your day with a glass of water to kickstart hydration after a night's sleep.
6. Variety: Keep your breakfast options diverse to ensure a wide range of nutrients.

Now that we've covered the fundamentals of a healthy breakfast for weight loss, let's explore a selection of delicious and nutritious breakfast recipes that align with these principles.

1. Greek Yogurt Parfait
Ingredients:
- 1/2 cup Greek yogurt (unsweetened)
- 1/4 cup granola (low sugar)
- 1/2 cup mixed berries (strawberries, blueberries, raspberries)
- 1 tablespoon honey (optional)

Instructions:
1. In a glass or bowl, layer Greek yogurt, granola, and mixed berries.
2. Drizzle honey on top if desired.
3. Enjoy your protein-packed and antioxidant-rich parfait.

2. Veggie Omelette
Ingredients:
- 2 large eggs
- 1/4 cup diced bell peppers
- 1/4 cup diced tomatoes
- 1/4 cup chopped spinach
- 1/4 cup diced onions
- Salt and pepper to taste
- Cooking spray or olive oil for the pan

Instructions:
1. Whisk the eggs in a bowl and season with salt and pepper.
2. Heat a non-stick skillet over medium heat and lightly coat it with cooking spray or olive oil.
3. Add the diced vegetables to the pan and sauté for a few minutes until they soften.
4. Pour the whisked eggs over the vegetables and let them cook, occasionally lifting the edges to allow uncooked egg to flow underneath.
5. Once the omelette is mostly set, carefully flip it in half to create a semi-circle shape.
6. Cook for another minute or so until fully set and lightly golden.

7. Slide it onto a plate and enjoy your vegetable-packed omelette.

3. Overnight Oats
Ingredients:
- 1/2 cup rolled oats
- 1/2 cup unsweetened almond milk (or your choice of milk)
- 1 tablespoon chia seeds
- 1/2 teaspoon vanilla extract
- 1/2 cup diced mango (or any fruit of your choice)
- 1 tablespoon chopped nuts (e.g., almonds, walnuts)
- 1 teaspoon honey or maple syrup (optional)

Instructions:
1. In a jar or container, combine rolled oats, almond milk, chia seeds, and vanilla extract. Stir well.
2. Add diced mango (or your chosen fruit) and chopped nuts on top.
3. Seal the container and refrigerate overnight.
4. In the morning, give it a good stir, and add a drizzle of honey or maple syrup if desired.
5. Enjoy your creamy and fiber-rich overnight oats.

4. Avocado Toast with Poached Egg
Ingredients:
- 1 slice whole-grain bread
- 1/2 ripe avocado
- 1 large egg
- Salt and pepper to taste
- Optional toppings: sliced tomatoes, red pepper flakes, or a sprinkle of feta cheese

Instructions:
1. Toast the whole-grain bread until it reaches your desired level of crispiness.
2. While the bread is toasting, mash the ripe avocado in a bowl and season with salt and pepper.
3. Poach the egg by bringing a small pot of water to a simmer. Add a splash of vinegar. Carefully crack the egg into a small cup and gently slide it into the simmering water. Poach for about 3-4 minutes or until the white is set but the yolk is still runny.

4. Remove the poached egg with a slotted spoon and drain any excess water.

5. Spread the mashed avocado on the toasted bread, and place the poached egg on top.

6. Add optional toppings if desired.

7. Savor your creamy avocado toast with a perfectly runny yolk.

5. Spinach and Mushroom Breakfast Quesadilla

Ingredients:
- 2 small whole-grain tortillas
- 1/2 cup chopped spinach
- 1/4 cup sliced mushrooms
- 2 large eggs
- 1/4 cup shredded low-fat cheese
- Salt and pepper to taste
- Cooking spray or olive oil for the pan

Instructions:
1. In a skillet, sauté the sliced mushrooms until they release moisture and turn golden brown. Add chopped spinach and continue to cook until wilted. Season with salt and pepper.

2. In a separate bowl, whisk the eggs and season with salt and pepper.

3. Heat a separate non-stick skillet over medium heat and lightly coat it with cooking spray or olive oil.

4. Pour half of the whisked eggs into the skillet and cook until set, gently lifting the edges to allow the uncooked egg to flow underneath.

5. Place one tortilla on top of the cooked eggs in the skillet.

6. Spread the sautéed mushrooms and spinach mixture on top of the tortilla.

7. Sprinkle shredded cheese over the veggies.

8. Place the second tortilla on top and press down gently.

9. Carefully flip the quesadilla to cook the other side until golden brown and the cheese is melted.

10. Slide it onto a plate, cut it into wedges, and enjoy your protein-packed breakfast quesadilla.

6. Peanut Butter Banana Smoothie
Ingredients:
- 1 ripe banana
- 1 tablespoon natural peanut butter
- 1/2 cup Greek yogurt (unsweetened)
- 1/2 cup unsweetened almond milk (or your choice of milk)
- 1 tablespoon honey (optional)
- Ice cubes (optional)

Instructions:
1. In a blender, combine the ripe banana, natural peanut butter, Greek yogurt, and almond milk.
2. Add honey for sweetness if desired.
3. If you prefer a colder smoothie, add a handful of ice cubes.
4. Blend until smooth and creamy.
5. Pour into a glass and enjoy your protein-rich and satisfying peanut butter banana smoothie.

7. Breakfast Burrito Bowl
Ingredients:
- 1/2 cup cooked quinoa
- 1/4 cup black beans (canned, drained, and rinsed)
- 1/4 cup diced tomatoes
- 1/4 cup diced bell peppers
- 1/4 cup diced avocado
- 1 large egg
- Salsa for drizzling
- Chopped cilantro for garnish
- Salt and pepper to taste
- Cooking spray or olive oil for the pan

Instructions:
1. In a skillet, sauté the diced bell peppers until they soften. Add diced tomatoes and black beans and cook until heated through. Season with salt and pepper.
2. While the veggies are cooking, prepare a sunny-side-up egg in a separate skillet.
3. In a bowl, assemble your breakfast burrito bowl by layering cooked quinoa, the sautéed veggie and bean mixture, diced avocado, and the sunny-side-up egg on top.

4. Drizzle with salsa and garnish with chopped cilantro.
5. Dive into your protein-packed and fiber-rich breakfast burrito bowl.

8. Cottage Cheese Pancakes
Ingredients:
- 1/2 cup low-fat cottage cheese

- 2 large eggs
- 1/4 cup rolled oats
- 1/4 teaspoon baking powder
- 1/4 teaspoon vanilla extract
- Cooking spray or olive oil for the pan
- Fresh berries for topping (e.g., strawberries, blueberries)

Instructions:
1. In a blender, combine low-fat cottage cheese, eggs, rolled oats, baking powder, and vanilla extract. Blend until smooth.
2. Heat a non-stick skillet over medium heat and lightly coat it with cooking spray or olive oil.
3. Pour small amounts of the pancake batter onto the skillet to create pancakes.
4. Cook until bubbles form on the surface, then flip and cook until golden brown on both sides.
5. Serve with fresh berries for a protein-packed and satisfying breakfast.

9. Smashed Avocado and Tomato Toast
Ingredients:
- 1 slice whole-grain bread
- 1/2 ripe avocado
- 1/2 cup diced tomatoes
- 1 teaspoon olive oil
- Salt and pepper to taste
- Optional toppings: sliced red onion, a sprinkle of feta cheese, or a drizzle of balsamic glaze

Instructions:
1. Toast the whole-grain bread until it reaches your desired level of crispiness.

2. While the bread is toasting, mash the ripe avocado in a bowl and season with salt and pepper.

3. In a separate bowl, combine diced tomatoes and olive oil, and season with salt and pepper.

4. Spread the mashed avocado on the toasted bread.

5. Top with the tomato mixture and add optional toppings if desired.

6. Enjoy your smashed avocado and tomato toast, packed with healthy fats and fresh flavors.

10. Chia Seed Pudding

Ingredients:
- 2 tablespoons chia seeds
- 1/2 cup unsweetened almond milk (or your choice of milk)
- 1/4 teaspoon vanilla extract
- 1/2 cup sliced strawberries
- 1 tablespoon chopped nuts (e.g., almonds, walnuts)
- 1 teaspoon honey (optional)

Instructions:
1. In a jar or container, combine chia seeds, almond milk, and vanilla extract. Stir well.

2. Seal the container and refrigerate for at least two hours or overnight until the mixture thickens into pudding-like consistency.

3. In the morning, give it a good stir, and add sliced strawberries and chopped nuts on top.

4. Drizzle with honey for sweetness if desired.

5. Enjoy your fiber-rich and omega-3-packed chia seed pudding.

11. Spinach and Feta Breakfast Wrap

Ingredients:
- 1 whole-grain tortilla
- 2 large eggs
- 1/2 cup chopped spinach
- 2 tablespoons crumbled feta cheese
- Salt and pepper to taste
- Cooking spray or olive oil for the pan

Instructions:
1. Heat a non-stick skillet over medium heat and lightly coat it with cooking spray or olive oil.
2. Whisk the eggs in a bowl and season with salt and pepper.
3. Add the chopped spinach to the skillet and sauté until wilted.
4. Pour the whisked eggs over the spinach and cook, occasionally lifting the edges to allow the uncooked egg to flow underneath.
5. Sprinkle crumbled feta cheese on top of the eggs.
6. Once the eggs are fully set, place the cooked mixture in the center of the whole-grain tortilla.
7. Fold the sides of the tortilla over the eggs to create a wrap.
8. Enjoy your protein-packed spinach and feta breakfast wrap.

12. Apple Cinnamon Oatmeal

Ingredients:
- 1/2 cup rolled oats
- 1 cup water
- 1/2 apple, diced
- 1/2 teaspoon ground cinnamon
- 1 tablespoon chopped nuts (e.g., almonds, pecans)
- 1 teaspoon honey or maple syrup (optional)

Instructions:
1. In a saucepan, bring water to a boil.
2. Stir in rolled oats and diced apple. Reduce heat to a simmer.
3. Add ground cinnamon and cook, stirring occasionally, until the oats are tender and the mixture has thickened.
4. Remove from heat and transfer to a bowl.
5. Top with chopped nuts and drizzle with honey or maple syrup if desired.
6. Enjoy your comforting and fiber-rich apple cinnamon oatmeal.

13. Berry Protein Smoothie Bowl

Ingredients:
- 1/2 cup frozen mixed berries (strawberries, blueberries, raspberries)
- 1/2 cup Greek yogurt (unsweetened)
- 1/4 cup unsweetened almond milk (or your choice of milk)
- 1 scoop of your favorite protein powder (vanilla or berry flavor)

- Toppings: sliced banana, chia seeds, granola, and fresh berries

Instructions:
1. In a blender, combine frozen mixed berries, Greek yogurt, almond milk, and protein powder.
2. Blend until smooth and creamy.
3. Pour the smoothie into a bowl.
4. Top with sliced banana, chia seeds, granola, and fresh berries.
5. Enjoy your protein-packed and antioxidant-rich smoothie bowl.

14. Sweet Potato and Black Bean Breakfast Bowl
Ingredients:
- 1 small sweet potato, peeled and cubed
- 1/4 cup black beans (canned, drained, and rinsed)

- 1/4 cup diced bell peppers
- 1/4 cup diced red onion
- 1 large egg
- 1 teaspoon olive oil
- Salt and pepper to taste
- Optional toppings: salsa, sliced avocado, chopped cilantro

Instructions:
1. Preheat your oven to 400°F (200°C).
2. Toss the cubed sweet potato with olive oil, salt, and pepper, and spread them on a baking sheet. Roast for about 20-25 minutes or until they are tender and lightly browned.
3. While the sweet potatoes are roasting, sauté the diced bell peppers and red onion in a skillet until softened.
4. Add black beans to the skillet and cook until heated through. Season with salt and pepper.
5. In a separate skillet, prepare a sunny-side-up egg.
6. Assemble your breakfast bowl by placing roasted sweet potatoes, sautéed veggies, and the sunny-side-up egg in a bowl.
7. Add optional toppings if desired.
8. Enjoy your fiber-rich and protein-packed sweet potato and black bean breakfast bowl.

15. Green Smoothie

Ingredients:
- 1 cup fresh spinach
- 1/2 ripe banana
- 1/2 cup diced pineapple (fresh or frozen)
- 1/2 cup unsweetened coconut water (or your choice of milk)
- 1 tablespoon chia seeds
- Optional: a drizzle of honey for sweetness

Instructions:
1. In a blender, combine fresh spinach, ripe banana, diced pineapple, coconut water, and chia seeds.
2. Add honey for sweetness if desired.
3. Blend until smooth and vibrant.
4. Pour into a glass and enjoy your nutrient-packed green smoothie. These delicious and nutritious breakfast recipes offer a wide range of options to keep your mornings exciting while supporting your weight loss goals. Remember to personalize these recipes to suit your taste preferences and dietary needs. Experiment with different ingredients and combinations to discover your favorite breakfast creations. In addition to these recipes, it's essential to stay hydrated throughout the morning by drinking water, herbal tea, or a low-calorie beverage of your choice. Hydration is a key element in maintaining overall health and supporting your weight loss journey. As you continue your weight loss journey, keep in mind that consistency, portion control, and mindful eating are crucial factors in achieving and maintaining your goals. Breakfast is just one piece of the puzzle, and your overall dietary choices and lifestyle play significant roles in your success. Start your mornings with intention and nourishment, and you'll find that making smart breakfast choices can set the stage for a healthier and happier you. Your journey to weight loss is a continuous process, and by incorporating these nutritious breakfast options, you're taking significant steps toward a healthier, more vibrant you. Enjoy your breakfasts, savor every bite, and celebrate the positive impact they have on your weight loss journey.

Lunch Recipes

Delicious and Nutritious Lunch Recipes for Your Weight Loss Journey

Lunchtime offers a fantastic opportunity to refuel your body and keep your energy levels steady throughout the day. When you're on a weight loss journey, making thoughtful and satisfying lunch choices is essential to help you stay on track towards your goals. In this comprehensive guide, we will explore the principles of a healthy lunch, the benefits it offers for weight loss, and a variety of delectable and nutritious lunch recipes that will keep you energized and satisfied. A well-balanced lunch is a vital component of your weight loss strategy, offering numerous benefits that go beyond satisfying your hunger. It provides a source of sustained energy that helps you power through the remainder of your day, preventing the mid-afternoon energy slump that often leads to unhealthy snacking or overeating. A balanced lunch supports your metabolism by contributing to stable blood sugar levels. This, in turn, can help prevent excessive calorie consumption later in the day, as erratic blood sugar levels can trigger cravings and impulsive eating. The impact of a nutritious lunch extends to cognitive function as well. By nourishing your body with the right combination of nutrients, you can stay alert, focused, and productive throughout the afternoon, making it easier to resist temptations and stick to your weight loss goals. Additionally, a well-balanced lunch can positively affect your mood and overall sense of well-being. Nutrient-rich foods can have a direct impact on your brain chemistry, potentially reducing cravings for sugary or high-calorie snacks that provide short-lived satisfaction but ultimately hinder your weight loss efforts. Lunch presents an excellent opportunity to increase your nutrient intake. By including a variety of vegetables, lean proteins, whole grains, and other nutrient-dense foods in your lunchtime meal, you ensure that your body receives the essential vitamins, minerals, fiber, and other nutrients necessary for optimal health. Finally, a well-balanced lunch is a cornerstone of your weight loss strategy, offering sustained energy, metabolic support, enhanced focus, improved mood, and increased nutrient intake. By making mindful choices at lunchtime, you set yourself up for success in managing your weight and overall well-being.

Principles of a Healthy Lunch for Weight Loss
Creating a healthy and weight-loss-friendly lunch involves adhering to these principles:
1. Protein-Rich: Include a lean source of protein like chicken, turkey, tofu, beans, or legumes to help keep you full and maintain muscle mass.
2. Fiber-Packed: Incorporate fiber-rich foods such as whole grains, vegetables, and legumes to promote satiety and digestive health.
3. Good Fats: Opt for sources of healthy fats like avocado, nuts, and olive oil, which contribute to feelings of fullness and support overall health.
4. Portion Control: Be mindful of portion sizes to avoid overeating. Pay attention to your body's hunger and fullness cues.
5. Variety: Keep your lunches diverse to ensure a wide range of nutrients and flavors.

Now that we've covered the fundamentals of a healthy lunch for weight loss, let's explore a selection of delicious and nutritious lunch recipes that align with these principles.

1. Grilled Chicken Salad
Ingredients:
- 4 oz grilled chicken breast, sliced
- 2 cups mixed greens (e.g., spinach, arugula, romaine)
- 1/2 cup cherry tomatoes, halved
- 1/4 cucumber, sliced
- 1/4 red onion, thinly sliced
- 1/4 cup sliced bell peppers
- 2 tablespoons balsamic vinaigrette dressing (reduced-fat)

Instructions:
1. In a large bowl, combine the mixed greens, cherry tomatoes, cucumber, red onion, and bell peppers.
2. Top the salad with the grilled chicken slices.
3. Drizzle with balsamic vinaigrette dressing.
4. Toss to combine and enjoy your protein-packed and fiber-rich grilled chicken salad.

2. Quinoa and Chickpea Bowl

Ingredients:
- 1/2 cup cooked quinoa
- 1/2 cup canned chickpeas, drained and rinsed
- 1/2 cup diced cucumber
- 1/2 cup diced bell peppers
- 1/4 cup diced red onion
- 2 tablespoons feta cheese (reduced-fat)
- 1 tablespoon olive oil
- 1 tablespoon lemon juice
- Salt and pepper to taste

Instructions:
1. In a bowl, combine cooked quinoa, chickpeas, cucumber, bell peppers, red onion, and feta cheese.
2. In a separate small bowl, whisk together olive oil and lemon juice.
3. Drizzle the dressing over the quinoa and chickpea mixture.
4. Season with salt and pepper to taste.
5. Toss to combine, and enjoy your protein-packed and fiber-rich quinoa and chickpea bowl.

3. Turkey and Avocado Wrap

Ingredients:
- 4 oz lean turkey breast slices
- 1 whole-grain tortilla
- 1/4 avocado, sliced
- 1/2 cup mixed greens
- 1 tablespoon Greek yogurt (plain, low-fat)
- Mustard or your favorite healthy condiment for flavor
- Optional toppings: sliced tomatoes, cucumber, or red onion

Instructions:
1. Lay the whole-grain tortilla flat on a clean surface.
2. Spread Greek yogurt and your preferred condiment evenly over the tortilla.
3. Layer turkey breast slices, avocado slices, mixed greens, and any optional toppings.
4. Roll the tortilla tightly, tucking in the sides as you go.

5. Slice the wrap in half and enjoy your protein-packed and fiber-rich turkey and avocado wrap.

4. Lentil and Vegetable Soup
Ingredients:
- 1 cup cooked brown or green lentils
- 2 cups mixed vegetables (e.g., carrots, celery, zucchini)
- 1/2 cup diced onion
- 2 cloves garlic, minced
- 4 cups low-sodium vegetable broth
- 1 teaspoon olive oil
- 1/2 teaspoon dried thyme
- Salt and pepper to taste

Instructions:
1. In a large pot, heat olive oil over medium heat.
2. Add diced onion and minced garlic and sauté until fragrant and translucent.
3. Add mixed vegetables and cook for a few minutes until slightly softened.
4. Pour in vegetable broth and add cooked lentils and dried thyme.
5. Bring the soup to a boil, then reduce heat and let it simmer for about 15-20 minutes or until the vegetables are tender.
6. Season with salt and pepper to taste.
7. Ladle the lentil and vegetable soup into a bowl and savor the fiber-rich and protein-packed goodness.

5. Greek Quinoa Salad
Ingredients:
- 1 cup cooked quinoa
- 1/2 cup diced cucumber
- 1/2 cup cherry tomatoes, halved
- 1/4 cup diced red onion
- 1/4 cup chopped fresh parsley
- 2 tablespoons crumbled feta cheese (reduced-fat)
- 1 tablespoon Kalamata olives, pitted and sliced
- 1 tablespoon olive oil
- 1 tablespoon lemon juice
- Salt and pepper to taste

Instructions:
1. In a large bowl, combine cooked quinoa, cucumber, cherry tomatoes, red onion, parsley, feta cheese, and Kalamata olives.
2. In a small bowl, whisk together olive oil and lemon juice.
3. Drizzle the dressing over the quinoa salad.
4. Season with salt and pepper to taste.
5. Toss to combine and enjoy your protein-packed and fiber-rich Greek quinoa salad.

6. Tofu and Vegetable Stir-Fry
Ingredients:
- 4 oz firm tofu, cubed
- 1 cup mixed vegetables (e.g., broccoli, bell peppers, snap peas)
- 1/4 cup sliced mushrooms
- 1/4 cup sliced carrots
- 2 cloves garlic, minced
- 1 tablespoon low-sodium soy sauce
- 1 tablespoon stir-fry sauce (low-sodium)
- 1 teaspoon sesame oil
- Cooking spray or olive oil for the pan
- Cooked brown rice or quinoa (optional, for serving)

Instructions:
1. Heat a non-stick skillet or wok over medium-high heat and lightly coat it with cooking spray or olive oil.
2. Add cubed tofu to the skillet and cook until it becomes lightly browned on all sides. Remove from the skillet and set aside.
3. In the same skillet, add minced garlic, mixed vegetables, mushrooms, and carrots. Stir-fry for a few minutes until the vegetables start to soften.
4. Return the cooked tofu to the skillet.
5. In a small bowl, combine low-sodium soy sauce, stir-fry sauce, and sesame oil. Pour the sauce over the tofu and vegetables.
6. Stir-fry for an additional 2-3 minutes until everything is well coated and heated through.
7. Serve your tofu and vegetable stir-fry over cooked brown rice or quinoa if desired, and enjoy your protein-packed and fiber-rich meal.

7. Salmon and Asparagus Foil Pack
Ingredients:
- 4 oz salmon fillet
- 8-10 spears of asparagus
- 1/4 cup sliced bell peppers
- 1/4 cup sliced red onion
- 1 tablespoon olive oil
- Lemon slices for garnish
- Salt and pepper to taste

Instructions:
1. Preheat your oven to 400°F (200°C).
2. Lay a large piece of aluminum foil on a baking sheet.
3. Place the salmon fillet in the center of the foil.
4. Arrange asparagus spears, bell peppers, and red onion slices around the salmon.
5. Drizzle olive oil over the salmon and vegetables.
6. Season with salt and pepper to taste.
7. Fold the foil over the salmon and vegetables to create a packet, sealing the edges.
8. Bake in the preheated oven for about 15-20 minutes or until the salmon is cooked through and flakes easily with a fork.
9. Garnish with lemon slices and savor your protein-packed and nutrient-rich salmon and asparagus foil pack.

8. Black Bean and Quinoa Salad
Ingredients:
- 1 cup cooked quinoa
- 1 cup canned black beans, drained and rinsed
- 1/2 cup corn kernels (fresh, frozen, or canned)
- 1/4 cup diced red bell pepper
- 1/4 cup diced green bell pepper
- 1/4 cup chopped cilantro
- 2 tablespoons lime juice
- 1 tablespoon olive oil
- Salt and pepper to taste
- Optional toppings: sliced avocado or a sprinkle of crumbled feta cheese

Instructions:

1. In a large bowl, combine cooked quinoa, black beans, corn kernels, red bell pepper, green bell pepper, and cilantro.
2. In a small bowl, whisk together lime juice and olive oil.
3. Drizzle the dressing over the quinoa and black bean salad.
4. Season with salt and pepper to taste.
5. Toss to combine and top with optional toppings if desired.
6. Enjoy your protein-packed and fiber-rich black bean and quinoa salad.

9. Egg Salad Lettuce Wraps

Ingredients:

- 2 large hard-boiled eggs, diced
- 1/4 cup diced celery
- 1/4 cup diced red onion
- 2 tablespoons Greek yogurt (plain, low-fat)
- 1 teaspoon Dijon mustard
- Salt and pepper to taste
- Romaine lettuce leaves for wrapping

Instructions:

1. In a bowl, combine diced hard-boiled eggs, diced celery, diced red onion, Greek yogurt, and Dijon mustard.
2. Season with salt and pepper to taste.
3. Mix until all ingredients are well combined.
4. Spoon the egg salad mixture onto romaine lettuce leaves.
5. Roll up the leaves to create lettuce wraps.
6. Enjoy your protein-packed and low-carb egg salad lettuce wraps.

10. Sweet Potato and Chickpea Salad

Ingredients:

- 1 small sweet potato, peeled and cubed
- 1/2 cup canned chickpeas, drained and rinsed
- 1/4 cup diced red onion
- 1/4 cup diced cucumber
- 1/4 cup chopped fresh parsley
- 2 tablespoons feta cheese (reduced-fat)
- 1 tablespoon olive oil
- 1 tablespoon lemon juice
- Salt and pepper to taste

Instructions:

1. Preheat your oven to 400°F (200°C).
2. Toss the cubed sweet potato with olive oil, salt, and pepper, and spread them on a baking sheet. Roast for about 20-25 minutes or until they are tender and lightly browned.
3. In a bowl, combine roasted sweet potatoes, chickpeas, red onion, cucumber, parsley, and feta cheese.
4. In a small bowl, whisk together lemon juice and olive oil.
5. Drizzle the dressing over the sweet potato and chickpea salad.
6. Season with salt and pepper to taste.
7. Toss to combine and enjoy your fiber-rich and protein-packed sweet potato and chickpea salad.

11. Caprese Stuffed Avocado

Ingredients:

- 1 ripe avocado, halved and pitted
- 1/2 cup cherry tomatoes, halved
- 2 tablespoons fresh basil leaves, torn
- 2 tablespoons mozzarella cheese (part-skim), diced
- 1 tablespoon balsamic glaze
- Salt and pepper to taste

Instructions:

1. Scoop out a bit of flesh from each avocado half to create a hollow space for the filling.
2. In a bowl, combine cherry tomatoes, torn basil leaves, and diced mozzarella cheese.
3. Season with salt and pepper to taste.
4. Spoon the tomato and cheese mixture into the hollowed-out avocados.
5. Drizzle with balsamic glaze.
6. Enjoy your nutrient-packed and satisfying Caprese stuffed avocado.

12. Spinach and Mushroom Quesadilla

Ingredients:

- 2 small whole-grain tortillas
- 1/2 cup sliced mushrooms
- 1 cup fresh spinach leaves
- 1/4 cup diced red onion

- 1/4 cup shredded low-fat cheese
- Salt and pepper to taste
- Cooking spray or olive oil for the pan

Instructions:
1. In a skillet, sauté the sliced mushrooms until they release moisture and turn golden brown. Add fresh spinach leaves and diced red onion and continue to cook until the spinach wilts. Season with salt and pepper.
2. Heat a separate non-stick skillet over medium heat and lightly coat it with cooking spray or olive oil.
3. Place one tortilla in the skillet and sprinkle shredded cheese evenly over the tortilla.
4. Spread the sautéed mushroom, spinach, and onion mixture on top of the cheese.
5. Place the second tortilla on top and press down gently.
6. Carefully flip the quesadilla to cook the other side until golden brown and the cheese is melted.
7. Slide it onto a plate, cut into wedges, and enjoy your protein-packed and veggie-filled spinach and mushroom quesadilla.

13. Chickpea and Avocado Salad
Ingredients:
- 1 cup canned chickpeas, drained and rinsed
- 1/2 ripe avocado, diced

- 1/4 cup diced red onion
- 1/4 cup diced cucumber
- 1/4 cup diced red bell pepper
- 2 tablespoons chopped fresh cilantro
- 2 tablespoons lime juice
- 1 tablespoon olive oil
- Salt and pepper to taste

Instructions:
1. In a bowl, combine chickpeas, diced avocado, diced red onion, diced cucumber, diced red bell pepper, and chopped cilantro.
2. In a small bowl, whisk together lime juice and olive oil.
3. Drizzle the dressing over the chickpea and avocado salad.
4. Season with salt and pepper to taste.

5. Toss to combine and enjoy your protein-packed and fiber-rich chickpea and avocado salad.

14. Turkey and Vegetable Stir-Fry
Ingredients:
- 4 oz lean ground turkey
- 1 cup mixed vegetables (e.g., broccoli, snap peas, carrots)
- 1/4 cup sliced mushrooms
- 1/4 cup diced bell peppers
- 1 clove garlic, minced
- 1 tablespoon low-sodium soy sauce
- 1 teaspoon olive oil
- Cooking spray or olive oil for the pan
- Cooked brown rice (optional, for serving)

Instructions:
1. Heat a non-stick skillet or wok over medium-high heat and lightly coat it with cooking spray or olive oil.
2. Add lean ground turkey to the skillet and cook until it's no longer pink, breaking it into crumbles as it cooks. Remove from the skillet and set aside.
3. In the same skillet, add minced garlic, mixed vegetables, mushrooms, and bell peppers. Stir-fry for a few minutes until the vegetables start to soften.
4. Return the cooked turkey to the skillet.
5. In a small bowl, whisk together low-sodium soy sauce and olive oil. Pour the sauce over the turkey and vegetables.
6. Stir-fry for an additional 2-3 minutes until everything is well coated and heated through.
7. Serve your turkey and vegetable stir-fry over cooked brown rice if desired, and enjoy your protein-packed and fiber-rich meal.

15. Lentil and Spinach Salad
Ingredients:
- 1 cup cooked green or brown lentils
- 2 cups fresh spinach leaves
- 1/4 cup diced red onion
- 1/4 cup diced cucumber
- 1/4 cup diced red bell pepper
- 2 tablespoons crumbled feta cheese (reduced-fat)

- 1 tablespoon olive oil
- 1 tablespoon balsamic vinegar
- Salt and pepper to taste

Instructions:
1. In a large bowl, combine cooked lentils, fresh spinach leaves, diced red onion, diced cucumber, diced red bell pepper, and crumbled feta cheese.
2. In a small bowl, whisk together olive oil and balsamic vinegar.
3. Drizzle the dressing over the lentil and spinach salad.
4. Season with salt and pepper to taste.
5. Toss to combine and enjoy your protein-packed and fiber-rich lentil and spinach salad.

16. Turkey and Vegetable Lettuce Wraps
Ingredients:
- 4 oz lean ground turkey
- 1/2 cup diced bell peppers
- 1/2 cup diced zucchini
- 1/4 cup diced red onion
- 1 clove garlic, minced
- 2 tablespoons low-sodium soy sauce
- 1 tablespoon hoisin sauce
- Romaine lettuce leaves for wrapping

Instructions:
1. In a skillet, heat a small amount of olive oil over medium heat.
2. Add lean ground turkey to the skillet and cook until it's no longer pink, breaking it into crumbles as it cooks. Remove from the skillet and set aside.
3. In the same skillet, add minced garlic, diced bell peppers, diced zucchini, and diced red onion. Sauté until the vegetables are tender.
4. Return the cooked turkey to the skillet.
5. In a small bowl, combine low-sodium soy sauce and hoisin sauce. Pour the sauce mixture over the turkey and vegetables.
6. Stir to combine and cook for an additional 2-3 minutes.
7. Spoon the turkey and vegetable mixture onto romaine lettuce leaves to create lettuce wraps.
8. Enjoy your protein-packed and low-carb turkey and vegetable lettuce wraps.

17. Mediterranean Tuna Salad

Ingredients:

- 1 can (5 oz) tuna in water, drained
- 1/4 cup diced cucumber
- 1/4 cup diced cherry tomatoes
- 2 tablespoons diced red onion
- 2 tablespoons Kalamata olives, pitted and sliced
- 1 tablespoon chopped fresh parsley
- 1 tablespoon olive oil
- 1 tablespoon lemon juice
- Salt and pepper to taste
- Optional toppings: feta cheese crumbles or sliced avocado

Instructions:

1. In a bowl, combine drained tuna, diced cucumber, diced cherry tomatoes, diced red onion, Kalamata olives, and chopped fresh parsley.
2. In a small bowl, whisk together olive oil and lemon juice.
3. Drizzle the dressing over the tuna salad.
4. Season with salt and pepper to taste.
5. Toss to combine and top with optional toppings if desired.
6. Enjoy your protein-packed and Mediterranean-inspired tuna salad.

18. Pesto and Veggie Pasta Salad

Ingredients:

- 1 cup cooked whole-grain pasta (e.g., whole wheat, quinoa, or chickpea pasta)
- 1/2 cup cherry tomatoes, halved
- 1/2 cup diced cucumber
- 1/4 cup sliced black olives
- 2 tablespoons pesto sauce (store-bought or homemade)
- 1 tablespoon olive oil
- 1 tablespoon balsamic vinegar
- Salt and pepper to taste
- Optional toppings: grated Parmesan cheese or pine nuts

Instructions:

1. In a bowl, combine cooked pasta, cherry tomatoes, diced cucumber, and sliced black olives.

2. In a small bowl, whisk together pesto sauce, olive oil, and balsamic vinegar.
3. Drizzle the dressing over the pasta salad.
4. Season with salt and pepper to taste.
5. Toss to combine and top with optional toppings if desired.
6. Enjoy your fiber-rich and flavorful pesto and veggie pasta salad.

19. Asian-Inspired Tofu Salad
Ingredients:
- 4 oz firm tofu, cubed
- 2 cups mixed greens (e.g., lettuce, spinach, kale)
- 1/2 cup shredded carrots
- 1/4 cup sliced cucumber
- 1/4 cup sliced red bell pepper
- 2 tablespoons low-sodium soy sauce
- 1 tablespoon rice vinegar
- 1/2 teaspoon sesame oil
- Sesame seeds for garnish (optional)

Instructions:
1. In a non-stick skillet, heat a small amount of olive oil over medium-high heat.
2. Add cubed tofu to the skillet and cook until it becomes lightly browned on all sides. Remove from the skillet and set aside.
3. In a bowl, combine mixed greens, shredded carrots, sliced cucumber, and sliced red bell pepper.
4. Top the salad with cooked tofu cubes.
5. In a small bowl, whisk together low-sodium soy sauce, rice vinegar, and sesame oil.
6. Drizzle the dressing over the tofu and salad.
7. Garnish with sesame seeds if desired.
8. Enjoy your protein-packed and flavorful Asian-inspired tofu salad.

20. Shrimp and Quinoa Bowl
Ingredients:
- 4 oz cooked shrimp (peeled and deveined)
- 1/2 cup cooked quinoa
- 1/2 cup steamed broccoli florets
- 1/4 cup diced red bell pepper

- 1/4 cup diced cucumber
- 2 tablespoons chopped fresh cilantro
- 1 tablespoon olive oil
- 1 tablespoon lime juice
- Salt and pepper to taste

Instructions:
1. In a bowl, combine cooked shrimp, cooked quinoa, steamed broccoli florets, diced red bell pepper, diced cucumber, and chopped cilantro.
2. In a small bowl, whisk together olive oil and lime juice.
3. Drizzle the dressing over the shrimp and quinoa bowl.
4. Season with salt and pepper to taste.
5. Toss to combine and enjoy your protein-packed and nutrient-rich shrimp and quinoa bowl.

21. Veggie and Hummus Wrap
Ingredients:
- 1 whole-grain tortilla
- 1/4 cup hummus (your choice of flavor)
- 1/2 cup mixed greens
- 1/4 cup shredded carrots
- 1/4 cup sliced cucumber
- 1/4 cup diced bell peppers
- 1/4 cup sliced cherry tomatoes
- Optional toppings: feta cheese crumbles or sliced olives

Instructions:
1. Lay the whole-grain tortilla flat on a clean surface.
2. Spread hummus evenly over the tortilla.
3. Layer mixed greens, shredded carrots, sliced cucumber, diced bell peppers, and sliced cherry tomatoes on top of the hummus.
4. Add optional toppings if desired.
5. Roll up the tortilla tightly, tucking in the sides as you go.
6. Slice the wrap in half and enjoy your fiber-rich and nutrient-packed veggie and hummus wrap.

22. Cucumber and Tuna Salad
Ingredients:
- 1 can (5 oz) tuna in water, drained

- 1/2 cup diced cucumber
- 1/4 cup diced red onion
- 1/4 cup diced celery
- 2 tablespoons Greek yogurt (plain, low-fat)
- 1 tablespoon Dijon mustard
- 1 tablespoon fresh dill, chopped
- Salt and pepper to taste

Instructions:
1. In a bowl, combine drained tuna, diced cucumber, diced red onion, diced celery, Greek yogurt, Dijon mustard, and fresh dill.
2. Season with salt and pepper to taste.
3. Mix until all ingredients are well combined.
4. Enjoy your protein-packed and refreshing cucumber and tuna salad.

23. Pita Bread and Hummus Plate
Ingredients:
- 1 whole-grain pita bread, cut into wedges
- 1/4 cup hummus (your choice of flavor)
- 1/2 cup mixed baby carrots, cucumber slices, and cherry tomatoes
- Optional additions: olives, feta cheese, or sliced bell peppers

Instructions:
1. Arrange whole-grain pita bread wedges on a plate.
2. Serve with a side of hummus for dipping.
3. Enjoy your satisfying and crunchy pita bread and hummus plate, complete with fresh vegetables and optional additions for added flavor.

24. Spaghetti Squash Primavera
Ingredients:
- 1/2 small spaghetti squash, cooked and strands separated
- 1/2 cup mixed vegetables (e.g., broccoli, cherry tomatoes, bell peppers)
- 1/4 cup diced red onion
- 1 clove garlic, minced
- 1 tablespoon olive oil
- 2 tablespoons grated Parmesan cheese
- Salt and pepper to taste

Instructions:
1. Preheat your oven to 375°F (190°C).
2. Cut the spaghetti squash in half lengthwise and remove the seeds.
3. Place the squash halves cut side down on a baking sheet and roast in the preheated oven for about 30-40 minutes or until the squash flesh is tender and can be easily scraped into strands with a fork.
4. While the squash is roasting, heat olive oil in a skillet over medium heat.
5. Add diced red onion and minced garlic and sauté until fragrant and translucent.
6. Add mixed vegetables to the skillet and cook until they are tender-crisp.
7. Once the spaghetti squash is done, scrape the flesh into strands using a fork and place them in a bowl.
8. Top the spaghetti squash with the sautéed vegetables.
9. Sprinkle with grated Parmesan cheese.
10. Season with salt and pepper to taste.
11. Enjoy your low-carb and veggie-packed spaghetti squash primavera.

25. Chickpea and Veggie Stir-Fry

Ingredients:
- 1 cup cooked chickpeas (canned, drained, and rinsed)
- 1 cup mixed vegetables (e.g., broccoli, snap peas, bell peppers)
- 1/4 cup sliced mushrooms
- 1/4 cup diced red onion
- 1 clove garlic, minced
- 1 tablespoon low-sodium soy sauce
- 1 tablespoon stir-fry sauce (low-sodium)
- 1 teaspoon sesame oil
- Cooking spray or olive oil for the pan
- Cooked brown rice or quinoa (optional, for serving)

Instructions:
1. Heat a non-stick skillet or wok over medium-high heat and lightly coat it with cooking spray or olive oil.
2. Add cooked chickpeas to the skillet and cook for a few minutes until heated through.
3. Remove the chickpeas from the skillet and set them aside.

4. In the same skillet, add minced garlic, mixed vegetables, sliced mushrooms, and diced red onion. Stir-fry for a few minutes until the vegetables start to soften.
5. Return the cooked chickpeas to the skillet.
6. In a small bowl, combine low-sodium soy sauce, stir-fry sauce, and sesame oil. Pour the sauce over the chickpeas and vegetables.
7. Stir-fry for an additional 2-3 minutes until everything is well coated and heated through.
8. Serve your chickpea and vegetable stir-fry over cooked brown rice or quinoa if desired, and enjoy your protein-packed and fiber-rich meal.

26. Eggplant and Tomato Salad
Ingredients:
- 1 small eggplant, diced
- 1 cup cherry tomatoes, halved
- ¼ cup diced red onion
- 2 cloves garlic, minced
- 1/4 cup chopped fresh basil
- 2 tablespoons balsamic vinegar
- 1 tablespoon olive oil
- Salt and pepper to taste

Instructions:
1. Preheat your oven to 400°F (200°C).
2. Toss the diced eggplant with olive oil, salt, and pepper, and spread them on a baking sheet.
3. Roast the eggplant in the preheated oven for about 20-25 minutes or until they are tender and slightly browned.
4. In a bowl, combine roasted eggplant, cherry tomatoes, diced red onion, minced garlic, chopped fresh basil, balsamic vinegar, and olive oil.
5. Season with salt and pepper to taste.
6. Toss to combine and enjoy your flavorful and nutrient-rich eggplant and tomato salad.

27. Turkey and Quinoa Stuffed Bell Peppers
Ingredients:
- 2 large bell peppers, halved and seeds removed
- 4 oz lean ground turkey

- 1/2 cup cooked quinoa
- 1/4 cup diced tomatoes (canned or fresh)
- 1/4 cup black beans (canned, drained, and rinsed)
- 1/4 cup diced red onion
- 1/4 cup diced zucchini
- 1/4 teaspoon chili powder
- 1/4 teaspoon ground cumin
- Salt and pepper to taste
- 2 tablespoons shredded low-fat cheese (optional)

Instructions:

1. Preheat your oven to 350°F (175°C).
2. Place bell pepper halves in a baking dish.
3. In a skillet, cook lean ground turkey over medium heat until it's no longer pink, breaking it into crumbles as it cooks.
4. Add diced red onion and diced zucchini to the skillet and sauté until they are tender.
5. Stir in cooked quinoa, diced tomatoes, black beans, chili powder, ground cumin, salt, and pepper.
6. Fill each bell pepper half with the turkey and quinoa mixture.
7. If desired, sprinkle shredded low-fat cheese on top.
8. Cover the baking dish with foil and bake in the preheated oven for about 30-35 minutes or until the bell peppers are tender.
9. Enjoy your protein-packed and fiber-rich turkey and quinoa stuffed bell peppers.

28. Tomato and Mozzarella Salad

Ingredients:

- 1 cup cherry tomatoes, halved
- 1/2 cup diced cucumber
- 1/4 cup diced red onion
- 1/4 cup fresh mozzarella cheese, diced
- 2 tablespoons fresh basil leaves, torn
- 1 tablespoon balsamic vinegar
- 1 tablespoon olive oil
- Salt and pepper to taste

Instructions:

1. In a bowl, combine cherry tomatoes, diced cucumber, diced red onion, fresh mozzarella cheese, and torn basil leaves.

2. In a small bowl, whisk together balsamic vinegar and olive oil.
3. Drizzle the dressing over the tomato and mozzarella salad.
4. Season with salt and pepper to taste.
5. Toss to combine and enjoy your refreshing and flavorful tomato and mozzarella salad.

29. Chicken and Vegetable Kebabs

Ingredients:
- 4 oz boneless, skinless chicken breast, cut into chunks
- 1/2 cup bell pepper chunks (assorted colors)
- 1/2 cup zucchini chunks
- 1/4 cup red onion chunks
- 1/4 cup cherry tomatoes
- 1 tablespoon olive oil
- 1 teaspoon dried Italian seasoning
- Salt and pepper to taste

Instructions:
1. Preheat your grill to medium-high heat.
2. Thread the chicken and vegetable chunks onto skewers, alternating between the ingredients.
3. In a small bowl, whisk together olive oil, dried Italian seasoning, salt, and pepper.
4. Brush the kebabs with the olive oil mixture.
5. Grill the kebabs for about 8-10 minutes, turning occasionally, or until the chicken is cooked through and the vegetables are tender.
6. Remove from the grill and enjoy your protein-packed and veggie-filled chicken and vegetable kebabs.

30. Spinach and Feta Omelette

Ingredients:
- 2 large eggs
- 1 cup fresh spinach leaves
- 2 tablespoons crumbled feta cheese (reduced-fat)
- 1/4 cup diced tomatoes
- 1/4 cup diced red onion
- Cooking spray or olive oil for the pan
- Salt and pepper to taste

Instructions:
1. In a bowl, beat the eggs until well combined.
2. Heat a non-stick skillet over medium heat and lightly coat it with cooking spray or olive oil.
3. Pour the beaten eggs into the skillet.
4. Add fresh spinach leaves, crumbled feta cheese, diced tomatoes, and diced red onion on one half of the omelette.
5. Season with salt and pepper to taste.
6. Carefully fold the other half of the omelette over the filling.
7. Cook for a few minutes until the omelette is set.
8. Slide it onto a plate, slice, and enjoy your protein-packed and veggie-filled spinach and feta omelette.

These lunch recipes provide a variety of options to help you achieve your weight loss goals while still enjoying delicious and satisfying meals. Remember to combine them with a balanced diet, regular physical activity, and portion control for the best results on your weight loss journey. Enjoy your nutritious and tasty lunches!

Dinner Recipes

Certainly, let's explore a collection of flavorful and healthy dinner recipes that will support your weight loss goals. These meals are designed to be both nutritious and satisfying, making them perfect additions to your meal prep routine.

1. Grilled Chicken Breast with Quinoa and Steamed Broccoli

Ingredients:
- 4 oz boneless, skinless chicken breast
- 1/2 cup cooked quinoa
- 1 cup steamed broccoli florets
- 1 tablespoon olive oil
- Lemon juice for drizzling
- Salt and pepper to taste

Instructions:
1. Preheat your grill to medium-high heat.
2. Brush the chicken breast with olive oil and season with salt and pepper.

3. Grill the chicken for about 6-8 minutes per side or until it's cooked through and no longer pink in the center.
4. Serve the grilled chicken with cooked quinoa and steamed broccoli.
5. Drizzle with lemon juice for added flavor.
6. Enjoy your protein-packed and fiber-rich dinner.

2. Baked Salmon with Roasted Vegetables
Ingredients:
- 4 oz salmon fillet
- 1 cup mixed vegetables (e.g., bell peppers, zucchini, carrots)
- 1 tablespoon olive oil
- Lemon slices for garnish
- Salt and pepper to taste

Instructions:
1. Preheat your oven to 375°F (190°C).
2. Place the salmon fillet on a baking sheet.
3. Toss mixed vegetables with olive oil, salt, and pepper, and spread them on the same baking sheet.
4. Bake in the preheated oven for about 15-20 minutes or until the salmon is cooked through and flakes easily with a fork.
5. Garnish with lemon slices for a burst of citrus flavor.
6. Enjoy your protein-packed and nutrient-rich salmon dinner.

3. Lentil and Vegetable Stir-Fry
Ingredients:
- 1 cup cooked green or brown lentils
- 1 cup mixed vegetables (e.g., broccoli, snap peas, bell peppers)
- 1/4 cup sliced mushrooms
- 1/4 cup diced red onion
- 1 clove garlic, minced
- 1 tablespoon low-sodium soy sauce
- 1 tablespoon stir-fry sauce (low-sodium)
- 1 teaspoon sesame oil
- Cooking spray or olive oil for the pan
- Cooked brown rice (optional, for serving)

Instructions:
1. Heat a non-stick skillet or wok over medium-high heat and lightly coat it with cooking spray or olive oil.
2. Add cooked lentils to the skillet and stir-fry for a few minutes until heated through.
3. Remove the lentils from the skillet and set them aside.
4. In the same skillet, add minced garlic, mixed vegetables, sliced mushrooms, and diced red onion. Stir-fry for a few minutes until the vegetables start to soften.
5. Return the cooked lentils to the skillet.
6. In a small bowl, combine low-sodium soy sauce, stir-fry sauce, and sesame oil. Pour the sauce over the lentils and vegetables.
7. Stir-fry for an additional 2-3 minutes until everything is well coated and heated through.
8. Serve your lentil and vegetable stir-fry over cooked brown rice if desired, and enjoy your protein-packed and fiber-rich dinner.

4. Turkey and Spinach Stuffed Bell Peppers
Ingredients:
- 2 large bell peppers, halved and seeds removed
- 4 oz lean ground turkey
- 1 cup fresh spinach leaves, chopped
- 1/4 cup diced tomatoes (canned or fresh)
- 1/4 cup cooked quinoa
- 1/4 cup diced red onion
- 1/4 teaspoon chili powder
- 1/4 teaspoon ground cumin
- Salt and pepper to taste
- 2 tablespoons shredded low-fat cheese (optional)

Instructions:
1. Preheat your oven to 350°F (175°C).
2. Place bell pepper halves in a baking dish.
3. In a skillet, cook lean ground turkey over medium heat until it's no longer pink, breaking it into crumbles as it cooks.
4. Add chopped fresh spinach leaves to the skillet and cook until wilted.
5. Stir in diced tomatoes, cooked quinoa, diced red onion, chili powder, ground cumin, salt, and pepper.
6. Fill each bell pepper half with the turkey and spinach mixture.

7. If desired, sprinkle shredded low-fat cheese on top.
8. Cover the baking dish with foil and bake in the preheated oven for about 30-35 minutes or until the bell peppers are tender.
9. Enjoy your protein-packed and fiber-rich stuffed bell peppers.

5. Shrimp and Veggie Stir-Fry

Ingredients:
- 4 oz cooked shrimp (peeled and deveined)
- 1 cup mixed vegetables (e.g., broccoli, snap peas, bell peppers)
- 1/4 cup sliced mushrooms
- 1/4 cup diced red onion
- 1 clove garlic, minced
- 1 tablespoon low-sodium soy sauce
- 1 tablespoon stir-fry sauce (low-sodium)
- 1 teaspoon sesame oil
- Cooking spray or olive oil for the pan
- Cooked brown rice or quinoa (optional, for serving)

Instructions:
1. Heat a non-stick skillet or wok over medium-high heat and lightly coat it with cooking spray or olive oil.
2. Add cooked shrimp to the skillet and stir-fry for a few minutes until heated through.
3. Remove the shrimp from the skillet and set them aside.
4. In the same skillet, add minced garlic, mixed vegetables, sliced mushrooms, and diced red onion. Stir-fry for a few minutes until the vegetables start to soften.
5. Return the cooked shrimp to the skillet.
6. In a small bowl, combine low-sodium soy sauce, stir-fry sauce, and sesame oil. Pour the sauce over the shrimp and vegetables.
7. Stir-fry for an additional 2-3 minutes until everything is well coated and heated through.
8. Serve your shrimp and vegetable stir-fry over cooked brown rice or quinoa if desired, and enjoy your protein-packed and fiber-rich dinner.

6. Sweet Potato and Black Bean Bowl

Ingredients:
- 1 small sweet potato, peeled and cubed
- 1/2 cup canned black beans, drained and rinsed

- 1/4 cup diced red onion
- 1/4 cup diced red bell pepper
- 2 tablespoons chopped fresh cilantro
- 1 tablespoon olive oil
- 1 tablespoon lime juice
- Salt and pepper to taste
- Optional toppings: avocado slices or Greek yogurt

Instructions:
1. Preheat your oven to 400°F (200°C).
2. Toss sweet potato cubes with olive oil, salt, and pepper, and spread them on a baking sheet.
3. Roast the sweet potatoes in the preheated oven for about 20-25 minutes or until they are tender and slightly browned.
4. In a bowl, combine roasted sweet potatoes, black beans, diced red onion, diced red bell pepper, and chopped fresh cilantro.
5. In a small bowl, whisk together lime juice and olive oil.
6. Drizzle the dressing over the sweet potato and black bean bowl.
7. Season with salt and pepper to taste.
8. Top with optional toppings if desired.
9. Enjoy your fiber-rich and nutrient-packed dinner.

7. Teriyaki Tofu and Vegetable Stir-Fry
Ingredients:
- 4 oz extra-firm tofu, cubed
- 1 cup mixed vegetables (e.g., broccoli, snap peas, bell peppers)
- 1/4 cup sliced mushrooms
- 1/4 cup diced red onion
- 1 clove garlic, minced
- 2 tablespoons low-sodium teriyaki sauce
- 1 tablespoon sesame oil
- Cooking spray or olive oil for the pan
- Cooked brown rice (optional, for serving)

Instructions:
1. Heat a non-stick skillet or wok over medium-high heat and lightly coat it with cooking spray or olive oil.
2. Add cubed tofu to the skillet and cook until it becomes lightly browned on all sides. Remove from the skillet and set aside.

3. In the same skillet, add minced garlic, mixed vegetables, sliced mushrooms, and diced red onion. Stir-fry for a few minutes until the vegetables start to soften.
4. Return the cooked tofu to the skillet.
5. In a small bowl, whisk together low-sodium teriyaki sauce and sesame oil. Pour the sauce over the tofu and vegetables.
6. Stir-fry for an additional 2-3 minutes until everything is well coated and heated through.
7. Serve your teriyaki tofu and vegetable stir-fry over cooked brown rice if desired, and enjoy your protein-packed and flavorful dinner.

8. Mediterranean Chickpea Salad

Ingredients:
- 1 cup canned chickpeas, drained and rinsed
- 1/2 cup diced cucumber
- 1/4 cup diced cherry tomatoes
- 2 tablespoons diced red onion
- 2 tablespoons Kalamata olives, pitted and sliced
- 1 tablespoon chopped fresh parsley
- 1 tablespoon olive oil
- 1 tablespoon lemon juice
- Salt and pepper to taste
- Optional toppings: feta cheese crumbles or sliced avocado

Instructions:
1. In a bowl, combine drained chickpeas, diced cucumber, diced cherry tomatoes, diced red onion, Kalamata olives, and chopped fresh parsley.
2. In a small bowl, whisk together olive oil and lemon juice.
3. Drizzle the dressing over the chickpea salad.
4. Season with salt and pepper to taste.
5. Toss to combine and top with optional toppings if desired.
6. Enjoy your protein-packed and Mediterranean-inspired chickpea salad.

9. Pesto Zucchini Noodles

Ingredients:
- 2 medium zucchinis, spiralized into noodles
- 2 tablespoons pesto sauce (store-bought or homemade)

- 1 tablespoon olive oil
- 1 clove garlic, minced
- Cherry tomatoes, halved, for garnish
- Grated Parmesan cheese for garnish (optional)
- Salt and pepper to taste

Instructions:
1. In a skillet, heat olive oil over medium heat.
2. Add minced garlic and cook until fragrant.
3. Add zucchini noodles to the skillet and sauté for a few minutes until they start to soften.
4. Stir in pesto sauce and continue to cook for another minute.
5. Season with salt and pepper to taste.
6. Garnish with halved cherry tomatoes and grated Parmesan cheese if desired.
7. Enjoy your low-carb and flavorful pesto zucchini noodles.

10. Spaghetti Squash with Marinara Sauce

Ingredients:
- 1/2 small spaghetti squash, cooked and strands separated
- 1/2 cup marinara sauce (low-sodium, store-bought or homemade)
- 2 tablespoons grated Parmesan cheese
- Fresh basil leaves for garnish (optional)
- Salt and pepper to taste

Instructions:
1. Preheat your oven to 375°F (190°C).
2. Cut the spaghetti squash in half lengthwise and remove the seeds.
3. Place the squash halves cut side down on a baking sheet and roast in the preheated oven for about 30-40 minutes or until the squash flesh is tender and can be easily scraped into strands with a fork.
4. Once the spaghetti squash is done, scrape the flesh into strands using a fork and place them on a plate.
5. Heat the marinara sauce in a saucepan over medium heat until it's warmed through.
6. Pour the warm marinara sauce over the spaghetti squash.
7. Sprinkle with grated Parmesan cheese.
8. Season with salt and pepper to taste.
9. Garnish with fresh basil leaves if desired.

10. Enjoy your low-carb and veggie-packed spaghetti squash with marinara sauce.

11. Greek Salad with Grilled Chicken
Ingredients:
- 4 oz boneless, skinless chicken breast
- 1 cup mixed greens (e.g., lettuce, spinach, kale)
- 1/4 cup diced cucumber
- 1/4 cup diced cherry tomatoes
- 2 tablespoons diced red onion
- 2 tablespoons Kalamata olives, pitted and sliced
- 2 tablespoons crumbled feta cheese (reduced-fat)
- 1 tablespoon olive oil
- 1 tablespoon balsamic vinegar
- Salt and pepper to taste

Instructions:
1. Preheat your grill to medium-high heat.
2. Brush the chicken breast with olive oil and season with salt and pepper.
3. Grill the chicken for about 6-8 minutes per side or until it's cooked through and no longer pink in the center.
4. In a bowl, combine mixed greens, diced cucumber, diced cherry tomatoes, diced red onion, Kalamata olives, and crumbled feta cheese.
5. In a small bowl, whisk together olive oil and balsamic vinegar.
6. Drizzle the dressing over the salad.
7. Season with salt and pepper to taste.
8. Slice the grilled chicken breast and place it on top of the salad.
9. Enjoy your protein-packed and Mediterranean-inspired Greek salad with grilled chicken.

12. Tuna and White Bean Salad
Ingredients:
- 1 can (5 oz) tuna in water, drained
- 1 cup canned white beans (cannellini or Great Northern), drained and rinsed
- 1/4 cup diced red onion
- 1/4 cup diced cucumber
- 2 tablespoons chopped fresh parsley

- 2 tablespoons olive oil
- 1 tablespoon lemon juice
- Salt and pepper to taste

Instructions:
1. In a bowl, combine drained tuna, white beans, diced red onion, diced cucumber, chopped fresh parsley, olive oil, and lemon juice.
2. Season with salt and pepper to taste.
3. Mix until all ingredients are well combined.
4. Enjoy your protein-packed and refreshing tuna and white bean salad.
13. Quinoa and Black Bean Bowl

Ingredients:
- 1/2 cup cooked quinoa
- 1/2 cup canned black beans, drained and rinsed
- 1/4 cup diced red bell pepper
- 1/4 cup diced cherry tomatoes
- 1/4 cup diced red onion
- 1/4 cup fresh cilantro leaves
- 1 tablespoon olive oil
- 1 tablespoon lime juice
- Salt and pepper to taste

Instructions:
1. In a bowl, combine cooked quinoa, black beans, diced red bell pepper, diced cherry tomatoes, diced red onion, and fresh cilantro leaves.
2. In a small bowl, whisk together olive oil and lime juice.
3. Drizzle the dressing over the quinoa and black bean bowl.
4. Season with salt and pepper to taste.
5. Toss to combine and enjoy your protein-packed and nutrient-rich dinner.

14. Baked Chicken Thighs with Roasted Vegetables
Ingredients:
- 4 oz chicken thighs (bone-in, skinless)
- 1 cup mixed vegetables (e.g., carrots, broccoli, cauliflower)
- 1 tablespoon olive oil
- Rosemary and thyme for seasoning
- Salt and pepper to taste

Instructions:
1. Preheat your oven to 375°F (190°C).
2. Place the chicken thighs on a baking sheet.
3. Toss mixed vegetables with olive oil, rosemary, thyme, salt, and pepper, and spread them on the same baking sheet.
4. Bake in the preheated oven for about 25-30 minutes or until the chicken is cooked through and the vegetables are tender.
5. Enjoy your protein-packed and veggie-filled baked chicken thighs with roasted vegetables.

15. Veggie and Tofu Stir-Fry
Ingredients:
- 4 oz extra-firm tofu, cubed
- 1 cup mixed vegetables (e.g., broccoli, snap peas, bell peppers)
- 1/4 cup sliced mushrooms
- 1/4 cup diced red onion
- 1 clove garlic, minced
- 1 tablespoon low-sodium soy sauce
- 1 tablespoon stir-fry sauce (low-sodium)
- 1 teaspoon sesame oil
- Cooking spray or olive oil for the pan
- Cooked brown rice or quinoa (optional, for serving)

Instructions:
1. Heat a non-stick skillet or wok over medium-high heat and lightly coat it with cooking spray or olive oil.
2. Add cubed tofu to the skillet and cook until it becomes lightly browned on all sides. Remove from the skillet and set aside.
3. In the same skillet, add minced garlic, mixed vegetables, sliced mushrooms, and diced red onion. Stir-fry for a few minutes until the vegetables start to soften.
4. Return the cooked tofu to the skillet.
5. In a small bowl, combine low-sodium soy sauce, stir-fry sauce, and sesame oil. Pour the sauce over the tofu and vegetables.
6. Stir-fry for an additional 2-3 minutes until everything is well coated and heated through.
7. Serve your veggie and tofu stir-fry over cooked brown rice or quinoa if desired, and enjoy your protein-packed and flavorful dinner.

16. Caprese Stuffed Portobello Mushrooms

Ingredients:
- 2 large portobello mushrooms, stems removed
- 1/2 cup diced tomatoes
- 1/4 cup fresh mozzarella cheese, diced
- 2 tablespoons fresh basil leaves, torn
- 1 tablespoon balsamic vinegar
- 1 tablespoon olive oil
- Salt and pepper to taste

Instructions:
1. Preheat your oven to 375°F (190°C).
2. Place portobello mushrooms on a baking sheet.
3. In a bowl, combine diced tomatoes, fresh mozzarella cheese, torn basil leaves, balsamic vinegar, olive oil, salt, and pepper.
4. Fill each portobello mushroom cap with the tomato and mozzarella mixture.
5. Bake in the preheated oven for about 20-25 minutes or until the mushrooms are tender.
6. Enjoy your flavorful and nutrient-rich caprese stuffed portobello mushrooms.

17. Cilantro Lime Shrimp with Quinoa

Ingredients:
- 4 oz cooked shrimp (peeled and deveined)
- 1/2 cup cooked quinoa
- 1/4 cup diced red bell pepper
- 1/4 cup diced cherry tomatoes
- 2 tablespoons chopped fresh cilantro
- 1 tablespoon olive oil
- 1 tablespoon lime juice
- Salt and pepper to taste

Instructions:
1. In a bowl, combine cooked shrimp, cooked quinoa, diced red bell pepper, diced cherry tomatoes, and chopped cilantro.
2. In a small bowl, whisk together olive oil and lime juice.
3. Drizzle the dressing over the shrimp and quinoa.
4. Season with salt and pepper to taste.

5. Toss to combine and enjoy your protein-packed and flavorful shrimp with quinoa.

18. Butternut Squash and Spinach Salad
Ingredients:
- 1 cup roasted butternut squash cubes
- 1 cup fresh spinach leaves
- 2 tablespoons chopped pecans
- 2 tablespoons crumbled feta cheese (reduced-fat)
- 1 tablespoon olive oil
- 1 tablespoon balsamic vinegar
- Salt and pepper to taste

Instructions:
1. Toss roasted butternut squash cubes with olive oil, salt, and pepper.
2. In a bowl, combine fresh spinach leaves, chopped pecans, and crumbled feta cheese.
3. Place the roasted butternut squash on top of the spinach salad.
4. In a small bowl, whisk together balsamic vinegar and olive oil.
5. Drizzle the dressing over the salad.
6. Season with salt and pepper to taste.
7. Enjoy your nutrient-rich and flavorful butternut squash and spinach salad.

19. Eggplant Parmesan
Ingredients:
- 1 small eggplant, sliced into rounds
- 1/2 cup marinara sauce (low-sodium, store-bought or homemade)
- 1/4 cup grated Parmesan cheese
- 1/4 cup shredded mozzarella cheese (part-skim)
- Fresh basil leaves for garnish (optional)
- Salt and pepper to taste

Instructions:
1. Preheat your oven to 375°F (190°C).
2. Arrange eggplant slices on a baking sheet.
3. Spread marinara sauce on top of each eggplant slice.
4. Sprinkle with grated Parmesan cheese and shredded mozzarella cheese.

5. Season with salt and pepper to taste.
6. Bake in the preheated oven for about 15-20 minutes or until the eggplant is tender and the cheese is melted and bubbly.
7. Garnish with fresh basil leaves if desired.
8. Enjoy your flavorful and low-calorie eggplant Parmesan.

20. Asian-Inspired Salmon Bowl

Ingredients:
- 4 oz salmon fillet
- 1/2 cup cooked brown rice
- 1 cup mixed vegetables (e.g., broccoli, snow peas, carrots)
- 1 tablespoon low-sodium soy sauce
- 1 tablespoon rice vinegar
- 1 teaspoon sesame oil
- Sesame seeds for garnish (optional)
- Salt and pepper to taste

Instructions:
1. Preheat your oven to 375°F (190°C).
2. Place the salmon fillet on a baking sheet.
3. Season with salt and pepper to taste.
4. Bake in the preheated oven for about 15-20 minutes or until the salmon is cooked through and flakes easily with a fork.
5. In a bowl, combine cooked brown rice and mixed vegetables.
6. In a small bowl, whisk together low-sodium soy sauce, rice vinegar, and sesame oil.
7. Drizzle the sauce over the rice and vegetable mixture.
8. Top with baked salmon.
9. Garnish with sesame seeds if desired.
10. Enjoy your Asian-inspired salmon bowl, rich in protein and flavor.

These 20 dinner recipes cover a wide range of flavors, ingredients, and dietary preferences, ensuring you have plenty of options to choose from for your weight loss journey. Remember to balance your meals, practice portion control, and incorporate regular exercise for a holistic approach to weight management. Enjoy your delicious and nutritious dinners!

Snack Recipes

Snack Recipes for Healthy Weight Loss

Snacking can be a double-edged sword when it comes to weight management. On one hand, it can help curb hunger between meals and provide an energy boost. On the other hand, mindless snacking on unhealthy options can lead to excess calorie intake and hinder your weight loss goals. The key to successful snacking for weight loss is making smart choices and being mindful of portion sizes. In this section, we'll explore a variety of delicious and nutritious snack recipes that can support your weight loss journey.

The Importance of Healthy Snacking

Understanding the importance of healthy snacking is paramount before we explore our recipes, as it plays a pivotal role in aiding your weight loss journey. When approached thoughtfully, snacking can offer an array of valuable benefits. Firstly, it serves as a tool for hunger control, helping to ward off excessive hunger that often leads to overindulgence during main meals. When you're overly hungry, making sound food choices and practicing portion control becomes increasingly challenging. Healthy snacks also contribute to the maintenance of consistent energy levels throughout the day. This steady supply of energy ensures you remain alert and focused, particularly beneficial for those with busy schedules or those engaging in regular physical activity. Selecting snacks that strike a balance between carbohydrates, protein, and healthy fats can work to stabilize blood sugar levels. This stability, in turn, curbs cravings for sugary and high-calorie foods, facilitating healthier dietary choices. A lesser-known advantage of healthy snacking is its potential to boost metabolism. By consuming small, balanced snacks between meals, you keep your metabolism active. This means that your body continues to burn calories even during the intervals between your primary meals, contributing to overall calorie expenditure. Snacking presents an excellent opportunity to enrich your nutrient intake. Opting for nutrient-dense snacks allows you to introduce crucial vitamins, minerals, fiber, and antioxidants into your diet, fortifying your overall health and well-being. In essence, the art of healthy snacking, when approached consciously, emerges as a valuable asset in supporting your weight loss endeavors and promoting your overall health. Now that we understand the benefits of healthy snacking, let's explore a variety of snack recipes that are not only delicious but also supportive of your weight loss goals.

Nutty Banana Oatmeal

Ingredients:
- 1 medium ripe banana, mashed
- 1/2 cup rolled oats
- 1 tablespoon natural almond butter
- 1 tablespoon chopped walnuts
- 1/2 teaspoon ground cinnamon
- 1/4 teaspoon pure vanilla extract
- Pinch of salt

Instructions:
1. In a bowl, combine the mashed banana, almond butter, and vanilla extract.
2. Stir in the rolled oats, chopped walnuts, ground cinnamon, and a pinch of salt.
3. Mix until all ingredients are well combined.
4. Form the mixture into bite-sized balls and place them on a parchment-lined tray.
5. Freeze for about 30 minutes to set.
6. Enjoy your nutty banana oatmeal bites as a satisfying and energy-boosting snack.

Greek Yogurt Parfait

Ingredients:
- 1/2 cup Greek yogurt (plain, non-fat)
- 1/2 cup mixed berries (e.g., strawberries, blueberries, raspberries)
- 1 tablespoon honey or maple syrup
- 1/4 cup granola (choose a low-sugar option)

Instructions:
1. In a glass or bowl, start by layering half of the Greek yogurt.
2. Add half of the mixed berries on top of the yogurt layer.
3. Drizzle half of the honey or maple syrup over the berries.
4. Sprinkle half of the granola as the next layer.
5. Repeat the layers with the remaining ingredients.

6. Enjoy your creamy and fruity Greek yogurt parfait.

Hummus and Veggie Sticks
Ingredients:
- 1/4 cup hummus (store-bought or homemade)
- Assorted vegetable sticks (carrots, cucumber, bell peppers, celery)

Instructions:
1. Wash and cut the assorted vegetables into sticks.
2. Serve them with a side of hummus for dipping.
3. Enjoy a crunchy, fiber-rich, and protein-packed snack that's perfect for satisfying your midday cravings.

Cottage Cheese and Pineapple
Ingredients:
- 1/2 cup low-fat cottage cheese
- 1/2 cup fresh pineapple chunks (or canned pineapple in its juice)

Instructions:
1. Place the cottage cheese in a bowl.
2. Top it with fresh pineapple chunks.
3. Enjoy the creamy and sweet combination of cottage cheese and pineapple, rich in protein and vitamin C.

Spicy Roasted Chickpeas
Ingredients:
- 1 can (15 oz) chickpeas, drained and rinsed
- 1 tablespoon olive oil
- 1/2 teaspoon paprika
- 1/4 teaspoon cayenne pepper
- 1/4 teaspoon garlic powder
- Salt to taste

Instructions:
1. Preheat your oven to 400°F (200°C).
2. In a bowl, toss the chickpeas with olive oil, paprika, cayenne pepper, garlic powder, and a pinch of salt.
3. Spread the seasoned chickpeas on a baking sheet.
4. Roast in the preheated oven for about 25-30 minutes, shaking the pan occasionally, until they are crispy.

5. Let them cool before enjoying your spicy roasted chickpeas as a crunchy and protein-rich snack.

Apple Slices with Almond Butter
Ingredients:
- 1 medium apple, sliced
- 2 tablespoons natural almond butter

Instructions:
1. Slice the apple into thin wedges or rounds.
2. Dip each apple slice into almond butter.
3. Enjoy the crispness of apples paired with the creaminess of almond butter—a perfect balance of sweetness and healthy fats.

Hard-Boiled Eggs with Avocado
Ingredients:
- 2 hard-boiled eggs, sliced
- 1/2 ripe avocado, sliced
- Sprinkle of salt and pepper

Instructions:
1. Slice the hard-boiled eggs and avocado.
2. Arrange them on a plate and season with a sprinkle of salt and pepper.
3. Enjoy the combination of protein from the eggs and healthy fats from the avocado—a satisfying and nutrient-packed snack.

Mini Caprese Skewers
Ingredients:
- Cherry tomatoes
- Fresh mozzarella cheese balls
- Fresh basil leaves
- Balsamic glaze (store-bought or homemade)
- Toothpicks

Instructions:
1. Thread a cherry tomato, a mozzarella cheese ball, and a fresh basil leaf onto each toothpick.
2. Drizzle with balsamic glaze.
3. Enjoy these bite-sized caprese skewers as a flavorful and low-calorie snack.

Cucumber and Tuna Bites
Ingredients:
- 1 cucumber, sliced into rounds
- 1 can (5 oz) tuna in water, drained
- 1 tablespoon Greek yogurt (plain, non-fat)
- 1/2 teaspoon Dijon mustard
- Fresh dill for garnish (optional)
- Salt and pepper to taste

Instructions:
1. In a bowl, combine the drained tuna, Greek yogurt, Dijon mustard, salt, and pepper.
2. Place a small spoonful of the tuna mixture on each cucumber round.
3. Garnish with fresh dill if desired.
4. Enjoy these refreshing and protein-packed cucumber and tuna bites.

Berry and Nut Trail Mix
Ingredients:
- 1/4 cup mixed nuts (e.g., almonds, walnuts, cashews)
- 1/4 cup dried berries (e.g., cranberries, blueberries)
- 1/4 cup dark chocolate chips (optional)
- 1/4 cup whole-grain cereal (choose a low-sugar option)

Instructions:
1. In a bowl, mix together the mixed nuts, dried berries, dark chocolate chips (if using), and whole-grain cereal.
2. Portion the trail mix into small, snack-sized bags for convenient, on-the-go snacking.
3. Enjoy the combination of crunchy nuts, sweet berries, and a touch of chocolate for a satisfying snack.

Green Smoothie
Ingredients:
- 1 cup unsweetened almond milk (or any milk of your choice)
- 1 cup fresh spinach leaves
- 1/2 ripe banana
- 1/2 cup frozen berries (e.g., blueberries, strawberries)
- 1 tablespoon chia seeds

- 1/2 teaspoon honey or maple syrup (optional)

Instructions:
1. Place all the ingredients in a blender.
2. Blend until smooth and creamy.
3. Add honey or maple syrup for a touch of sweetness if desired.
4. Pour into a glass and enjoy your nutritious and green smoothie.

Edamame with Sea Salt
Ingredients:
- 1 cup edamame (frozen, steamed, and lightly salted)

Instructions:
1. Steam the frozen edamame according to the package instructions.
2. Sprinkle with sea salt.
3. Enjoy these protein-packed and lightly salted edamame beans as a satisfying snack.

DIY Popcorn
Ingredients:
- 1/4 cup popcorn kernels
- 1 tablespoon olive oil
- Nutritional yeast (optional, for a cheesy flavor)
- Seasonings of your choice (e.g., paprika, garlic powder, chili powder)

Instructions:
1. In a large pot, heat the olive oil over medium-high heat.
2. Add the popcorn kernels and cover with a lid.
3. Shake the pot occasionally to prevent burning.
4. Once the popping slows down, remove the pot from heat.
5. Sprinkle with nutritional yeast and your choice of seasonings.
6. Enjoy your homemade popcorn—a whole-grain, fiber-rich snack.

Sweet Potato Chips
Ingredients:
- 1 large sweet potato, thinly sliced
- 1 tablespoon olive oil
- 1/2 teaspoon paprika
- 1/4 teaspoon garlic powder

- Salt and pepper to taste

Instructions:
1. Preheat your oven to 400°F (200°C).
2. In a bowl, toss the sweet potato slices with olive oil, paprika, garlic powder, salt, and pepper.
3. Spread the seasoned sweet potato slices on a baking sheet.
4. Bake in the preheated oven for about 15-20 minutes or until they are crisp.
5. Let them cool before enjoying your homemade sweet potato chips as a crunchy and vitamin A-rich snack.

Frozen Grapes
Ingredients:
- Fresh grapes (any variety)

Instructions:
1. Wash and dry the grapes.
2. Place them in a single layer on a baking sheet.
3. Freeze for at least 2 hours.
4. Enjoy these naturally sweet and refreshing frozen grapes as a guilt-free snack.

Avocado and Salsa
Ingredients:
- 1/2 ripe avocado, sliced
- 2 tablespoons salsa (store-bought or homemade)
- Whole-grain crackers or rice cakes (optional)

Instructions:
1. Slice the ripe avocado.
2. Top the avocado slices with salsa.
3. Serve with whole-grain crackers or rice cakes if desired.
4. Enjoy the creamy avocado paired with the zesty salsa for a satisfying snack.

Mini Veggie Frittatas
Ingredients:
- Cooking spray or olive oil for the muffin tin
- 4 large eggs

- 1/4 cup diced bell peppers
- 1/4 cup diced onions
- 1/4 cup diced spinach or kale
- 1/4 cup diced tomatoes
- Salt and pepper to taste

Instructions:
1. Preheat your oven to 350°F (175°C).
2. Lightly grease a muffin tin with cooking spray or olive oil.
3. In a bowl, whisk the eggs and season with salt and pepper.
4. Divide the diced vegetables evenly among the muffin cups.
5. Pour the beaten eggs over the vegetables, filling each cup about two-thirds full.
6. Bake in the preheated oven for about 15-20 minutes or until the frittatas are set and slightly golden on top.
7. Let them cool before removing them from the muffin tin.
8. Enjoy these mini veggie frittatas as a protein-packed and portable snack.

Almond and Cherry Protein Balls
Ingredients:
- 1/2 cup dried cherries
- 1/2 cup almonds
- 1/4 cup rolled oats
- 2 tablespoons vanilla protein powder
- 1 tablespoon honey or maple syrup
- Pinch of salt

Instructions:
1. In a food processor, combine dried cherries, almonds, rolled oats, vanilla protein powder, honey or maple syrup, and a pinch of salt.
2. Pulse until the mixture comes together and forms a sticky dough.
3. Roll the dough into bite-sized balls.
4. Place them in the refrigerator to set for about 30 minutes.
5. Enjoy your almond and cherry protein balls as a satisfying and protein-rich snack.

Spinach and Feta Stuffed Mushrooms
Ingredients:
- 6 large mushroom caps, stems removed

- 1 cup fresh spinach leaves, chopped
- 1/4 cup crumbled feta cheese (reduced-fat)
- 1 clove garlic, minced
- 1 tablespoon olive oil
- Salt and pepper to taste

Instructions:
1. Preheat your oven to 350°F (175°C).
2. In a skillet, heat olive oil over medium heat.
3. Add minced garlic and sauté until fragrant.
4. Stir in chopped spinach and cook until wilted.
5. Remove from heat and let it cool slightly.
6. In a bowl, combine the cooked spinach and crumbled feta cheese.
7. Season with salt and pepper.
8. Fill each mushroom cap with the spinach and feta mixture.
9. Place them on a baking sheet.
10. Bake in the preheated oven for about 15-20 minutes or until the mushrooms are tender.
11. Enjoy your savory and low-calorie spinach and feta stuffed mushrooms.

Tzatziki and Veggie Dippers
Ingredients:
- 1/2 cup Greek yogurt (plain, non-fat)
- 1/2 cucumber, finely grated and drained
- 1 clove garlic, minced
- 1 tablespoon fresh dill, chopped
- Salt and pepper to taste
- Assorted vegetable dippers (e.g., carrot sticks, cucumber slices)

Instructions:
1. In a bowl, combine Greek yogurt, finely grated and drained cucumber, minced garlic, fresh dill, salt, and pepper.
2. Mix until well blended.
3. Serve the tzatziki sauce with assorted vegetable dippers.
4. Enjoy a creamy and refreshing dip with a variety of crunchy veggies.

Chocolate Banana Protein Smoothie
Ingredients:
- 1 cup unsweetened almond milk (or any milk of your choice)
- 1 medium ripe banana
- 1 scoop chocolate protein powder
- 1 tablespoon natural peanut butter
- 1/2 teaspoon unsweetened cocoa powder
- Ice cubes (optional)
- Honey or maple syrup for sweetness (optional)

Instructions:
1. Place all the ingredients in a blender.
2. Blend until smooth and creamy.
3. Add honey or maple syrup for sweetness if desired.
4. Pour into a glass and enjoy your indulgent yet nutritious chocolate banana protein smoothie.

Cinnamon Roasted Almonds
Ingredients:
- 1 cup raw almonds
- 1 tablespoon olive oil
- 1 tablespoon honey
- 1/2 teaspoon ground cinnamon
- Pinch of salt

Instructions:
1. Preheat your oven to 350°F (175°C).
2. In a bowl, mix the raw almonds with olive oil, honey, ground cinnamon, and a pinch of salt.
3. Spread the almonds on a baking sheet.
4. Roast in the preheated oven for about 10-15 minutes or until they are lightly toasted.
5. Let them cool before enjoying your sweet and crunchy cinnamon-roasted almonds.

Snacking doesn't have to sabotage your weight loss efforts. With these delicious and nutritious snack recipes, you can satisfy your cravings while supporting your health and wellness goals.

Remember to practice portion control and choose snacks that provide a balance of protein, fiber, and healthy fats. By making mindful snack choices, you can maintain energy levels, control hunger, and enjoy the journey toward a healthier you.

Chapter 4
Special Dietary Considerations

Special Dietary Considerations - Vegan and Vegetarian Meal Prep

Incorporating plant-based eating into your lifestyle offers numerous health benefits, from reducing the risk of chronic diseases to promoting sustainable food choices. Whether you're a committed vegan or simply exploring the world of vegetarianism, meal prepping can be a powerful tool to help you maintain a balanced, nutrient-rich diet. In this chapter, we'll delve into the art of vegan and vegetarian meal prepping, exploring its benefits, essential nutrients to consider, and providing you with a collection of delicious plant-based recipes.

The Benefits of Vegan and Vegetarian Meal Prep

1. Enhanced Nutrient Intake: A well-planned vegan or vegetarian diet can be rich in essential nutrients like fiber, vitamins, minerals, and antioxidants. Meal prepping allows you to consistently incorporate a variety of plant foods into your diet, ensuring a broad spectrum of nutrients.

2. Weight Management: Plant-based diets tend to be lower in calorie density, making them an excellent choice for weight management. Meal prepping enables you to control portion sizes and create balanced, satisfying meals that support your weight loss or maintenance goals.

3. Sustainability: Choosing plant-based foods reduces your environmental footprint. Meal prepping plant-based meals can further contribute to sustainability by minimizing food waste and reducing the need for single-use packaging.

4. Time Savings: Vegan and vegetarian meal prep can save you valuable time during the week. Having pre-made meals and snacks at your fingertips eliminates the need for daily cooking, making it easier to stick to your dietary goals.

Essential Nutrients for Vegans and Vegetarians

When following a vegan or vegetarian diet, it's important to pay attention to certain nutrients to ensure you're meeting your body's needs. Here are some key nutrients to focus on:

1. Protein: Plant-based sources of protein include beans, lentils, tofu, tempeh, edamame, quinoa, and nuts. Incorporate a variety of these protein-rich foods into your meals to meet your protein requirements.

2. Iron: Iron from plant-based sources (non-heme iron) is less readily absorbed by the body compared to iron from animal sources (heme iron). To enhance iron absorption, pair iron-rich foods with vitamin C sources like citrus fruits, strawberries, and bell peppers.

3. Vitamin B12: Vitamin B12 is primarily found in animal products, so vegans should consider fortified foods like plant-based milk, breakfast cereals, and nutritional yeast, or take a B12 supplement as recommended by a healthcare professional.

4. Calcium: Calcium-rich plant foods include fortified plant-based milk, leafy greens (like kale and collard greens), almonds, tahini, and fortified tofu. Ensure these foods are part of your meal prep to support bone health.

5. Omega-3 Fatty Acids: Sources of omega-3s for vegans and vegetarians include flaxseeds, chia seeds, walnuts, and hemp seeds. Incorporate these into your meal prep for heart and brain health.

Vegan and Vegetarian Meal Prep Tips

Efficient vegan and vegetarian meal prep is a cornerstone of maintaining a nutritious and satisfying plant-based diet. Here are some strategies to streamline your meal preparation:

1. Plan Balanced Meals: Craft your meals with a harmonious blend of plant-based protein sources, vibrant vegetables, whole grains, and nourishing fats. This thoughtful composition ensures you receive a comprehensive spectrum of essential nutrients for optimal well-being.

2. Batch Cook Staples: Simplify your weekly meal prep by preparing substantial batches of fundamental ingredients such as brown rice, quinoa, beans (like black beans and chickpeas), and versatile sauces like tomato sauce or pesto. These staples can serve as the foundation for various dishes throughout the week, saving you time and effort.

3. Experiment with Global Flavors: Infuse excitement and variety into your vegan and vegetarian meal prep by venturing into the realm of international cuisines. Embrace recipes from diverse culinary traditions, including Asian, Mediterranean, Mexican, and Indian, to tantalize your taste buds with a rich array of flavors and ingredients.

4. Utilize Mason Jar Salads: Elevate your salad game with the convenience of mason jar salads. Assemble your salads with the dressing at the bottom, followed by heartier elements like grains and beans, and top it off with leafy greens. When it's time to enjoy your meal, a simple shake of the jar ensures an even distribution of dressing, making it a practical and flavorful choice.

5. Prep Smart Snacks: Don't overlook the importance of healthy snacking in your vegan or vegetarian diet. Prepare a selection of wholesome plant-based snacks such as crisp veggie sticks paired with hummus, homemade granola bars, refreshing fruit salads, or guilt-free air-popped popcorn. These ready-to-go options ensure you have convenient and nutritious choices at hand whenever hunger strikes.

Incorporating these meal prep strategies into your vegan or vegetarian lifestyle will not only simplify your culinary endeavors but also enhance the diversity and richness of your plant-based diet, making it both enjoyable and sustainable.

Delicious Vegan and Vegetarian Meal Prep Recipes

1. Chickpea and Vegetable Stir-Fry
Ingredients:
- 1 can (15 oz) chickpeas, drained and rinsed
- 2 cups mixed vegetables (e.g., bell peppers, broccoli, snap peas)
- 2 cloves garlic, minced
- 2 tablespoons low-sodium soy sauce or tamari
- 1 tablespoon sesame oil
- 1 teaspoon grated ginger
- Cooked brown rice or quinoa

Instructions:
1. In a large skillet or wok, heat the sesame oil over medium-high heat.

2. Add minced garlic and grated ginger, sauté for about 30 seconds.
3. Add mixed vegetables and stir-fry for 5-7 minutes until they become tender-crisp.
4. Add chickpeas and soy sauce (or tamari), stir to combine, and cook for an additional 2-3 minutes.
5. Serve over cooked brown rice or quinoa for a protein-packed meal.

2. Lentil and Sweet Potato Curry
Ingredients:
- 1 cup dried green or brown lentils
- 2 large sweet potatoes, peeled and diced
- 1 can (14 oz) diced tomatoes
- 1 can (14 oz) coconut milk
- 2 tablespoons curry paste (adjust to taste)
- 1 onion, chopped
- 2 cloves garlic, minced
- 1 tablespoon olive oil
- Fresh cilantro for garnish
- Cooked basmati rice

Instructions:
1. Rinse the lentils and set them aside.
2. In a large pot, heat olive oil over medium heat.
3. Add chopped onion and minced garlic, sauté until translucent.
4. Stir in the curry paste and cook for 1-2 minutes.
5. Add diced sweet potatoes, lentils, diced tomatoes (with juice), and coconut milk.
6. Bring to a boil, then reduce the heat, cover, and simmer for about 25-30 minutes or until the sweet potatoes and lentils are tender.
7. Serve over cooked basmati rice, garnished with fresh cilantro.

3. Vegan Chickpea Salad Sandwich
Ingredients:
- 1 can (15 oz) chickpeas, drained and rinsed
- 1/4 cup vegan mayo
- 2 tablespoons Dijon mustard
- 1/2 cup diced celery
- 1/4 cup diced red onion

- 2 tablespoons chopped fresh dill (or 1 teaspoon dried dill)
- Salt and pepper to taste
- Whole-grain bread or wraps
- Lettuce, tomato, and avocado for sandwich filling

Instructions:

1. In a mixing bowl, mash the chickpeas with a fork or potato masher.

2. Add vegan mayo, Dijon mustard, diced celery, diced red onion, chopped dill, salt, and pepper. Mix until well combined.

3. Toast whole-grain bread or warm whole-grain wraps.

4. Assemble sandwiches or wraps with chickpea salad, lettuce, tomato, and avocado slices.

4. Vegan Quinoa and Black Bean Bowl

Ingredients:

- 1 cup quinoa, rinsed and drained
- 1 can (15 oz) black beans, drained and rinsed
- 1 cup corn kernels (fresh, frozen, or canned)
- 1 cup cherry tomatoes, halved
- 1/2 red onion, finely chopped
- 1/4 cup fresh cilantro, chopped
- Juice of 2 limes
- 1 tablespoon olive oil
- Salt and pepper to taste
- Avocado slices for garnish

Instructions:

1. Cook quinoa according to package instructions.

2. In a large bowl, combine cooked quinoa, black beans, corn kernels, cherry tomatoes, finely chopped red onion, and fresh cilantro.

3. In a small bowl, whisk together lime juice and olive oil. Season with salt and pepper.

4. Drizzle the dressing over the quinoa and bean mixture and toss to combine.

5. Garnish with avocado slices before serving.

5. Roasted Vegetable and Hummus Wrap

Ingredients:
- Assorted vegetables (e.g., bell peppers, zucchini, red onion, cherry tomatoes)
- Olive oil
- Salt and pepper
- Whole-grain wraps
- Hummus
- Fresh spinach or arugula

Instructions:
1. Preheat your oven to 400°F (200°C).
2. Slice the assorted vegetables into strips.
3. Toss the vegetables with olive oil, salt, and pepper.
4. Spread the vegetables evenly on a baking sheet and roast for about 20-25 minutes or until they are tender and slightly caramelized.
5. Spread hummus onto whole-grain wraps.
6. Add a handful of fresh spinach or arugula.
7. Top with roasted vegetables.
8. Roll up the wraps and enjoy your flavorful and satisfying meal.

Vegan and vegetarian meal prep opens the door to a world of delicious, nutritious, and sustainable eating. By planning balanced meals, paying attention to essential nutrients, and experimenting with diverse flavors, you can create a wide variety of plant-based dishes that support your health and well-being. Whether you're a seasoned vegan or just beginning your journey into plant-based eating, meal prepping can make the transition smoother and more enjoyable.

Gluten-Free Meal Prep

Gluten-free meal prep is a valuable tool for individuals with celiac disease, gluten sensitivity, or those who choose to follow a gluten-free diet for various health reasons. When done thoughtfully, gluten-free meal prep can ensure that you enjoy delicious, safe, and nutritious meals without the worry of gluten contamination. In this chapter, we'll explore the fundamentals of gluten-free meal prep, discuss the benefits, address potential challenges, and provide a collection of delectable gluten-free recipes to elevate your culinary experience.

Understanding Gluten and Gluten-Free Eating

What is Gluten?
Gluten is a protein found in wheat, barley, rye, and their derivatives. For individuals with celiac disease or non-celiac gluten sensitivity, consuming gluten-containing foods can trigger adverse reactions, ranging from digestive issues to autoimmune responses.

Benefits of a Gluten-Free Diet
- Relief from Symptoms: A gluten-free diet can alleviate symptoms for those with celiac disease, such as gastrointestinal discomfort, fatigue, and skin problems.
- Improved Digestion: Individuals with gluten sensitivity often experience improved digestion and reduced bloating and gas when eliminating gluten from their diet.
- Increased Nutrient Intake: Embracing gluten-free whole grains, like quinoa, rice, and buckwheat, can lead to a more diverse nutrient intake.

Gluten-Free Meal Prep Essentials
1. A Gluten-Free Kitchen: To avoid cross-contamination, maintain a dedicated gluten-free area in your kitchen. Use separate utensils, cutting boards, and cookware for gluten-free meal prep.
2. Gluten-Free Pantry Staples: Stock your pantry with gluten-free essentials like gluten-free flour blends, gluten-free soy sauce (tamari), gluten-free pasta, and certified gluten-free oats.
3. Fresh Produce and Whole Foods: Fruits, vegetables, lean proteins, dairy products (if tolerated), and naturally gluten-free grains (like quinoa and rice) are the foundation of your gluten-free meal prep.
4. Read Labels: Always read food labels carefully to identify hidden sources of gluten. Look for gluten-free certifications and familiarize yourself with gluten-containing ingredients.

Gluten-Free Meal Prep Tips
1. Plan Gluten-Free Meals: Design a meal plan that centers around naturally gluten-free foods. Embrace the beauty of whole, unprocessed ingredients to create safe and delicious meals.

2. Batch Cooking: Prepare gluten-free grains, proteins, and sauces in large quantities to use as the building blocks for multiple meals during the week.

3. Use Gluten-Free Substitutes: Experiment with gluten-free flours, such as almond flour, coconut flour, or chickpea flour, to recreate gluten-containing favorites like pancakes and baked goods.

4. Opt for Homemade Sauces: Create your gluten-free sauces, dressings, and marinades to ensure they are safe for your dietary needs.

Delectable Gluten-Free Meal Prep Recipes

1. Quinoa and Roasted Vegetable Salad

Ingredients:
- 1 cup quinoa, rinsed and drained
- Assorted vegetables (e.g., bell peppers, zucchini, cherry tomatoes)
- Olive oil
- Salt and pepper
- Fresh basil leaves, chopped
- Balsamic vinaigrette dressing (gluten-free)
- Optional: crumbled feta cheese (ensure it's gluten-free)

Instructions:
1. Cook quinoa according to package instructions.
2. Preheat your oven to 400°F (200°C).
3. Slice the assorted vegetables into strips.
4. Toss the vegetables with olive oil, salt, and pepper.
5. Spread the vegetables evenly on a baking sheet and roast for about 20-25 minutes or until they are tender and slightly caramelized.
6. In a large bowl, combine cooked quinoa, roasted vegetables, and chopped fresh basil.
7. Drizzle with gluten-free balsamic vinaigrette dressing and toss to combine.
8. If desired, top with crumbled feta cheese.
9. Divide the salad into meal prep containers for a hearty and satisfying gluten-free lunch.

2. Grilled Chicken with Lemon-Herb Quinoa

Ingredients:
- 4 boneless, skinless chicken breasts
- Olive oil
- Salt and pepper
- 1 cup quinoa, rinsed and drained
- Zest and juice of 2 lemons
- Fresh parsley, chopped
- Fresh dill, chopped
- Gluten-free chicken broth (for cooking quinoa)

Instructions:
1. Preheat your grill to medium-high heat.
2. Brush chicken breasts with olive oil and season with salt and pepper.
3. Grill chicken for about 6-8 minutes per side or until cooked through.
4. While the chicken is grilling, cook quinoa in gluten-free chicken broth according to package instructions.
5. In a bowl, combine cooked quinoa, lemon zest, lemon juice, chopped fresh parsley, and chopped fresh dill.
6. Season with salt and pepper to taste.
7. Divide the lemon-herb quinoa and grilled chicken into meal prep containers for a delightful gluten-free dinner.

3. Gluten-Free Veggie Wrap

Ingredients:
- Gluten-free tortillas or wraps
- Hummus (ensure it's gluten-free)
- Sliced cucumbers
- Sliced bell peppers
- Sliced carrots
- Baby spinach leaves
- Sliced cooked chicken or chickpeas (for added protein)
- Gluten-free balsamic vinaigrette dressing

Instructions:
1. Lay out a gluten-free tortilla or wrap.
2. Spread a generous layer of gluten-free hummus over the tortilla.

3. Layer sliced cucumbers, bell peppers, carrots, baby spinach leaves, and your choice of sliced cooked chicken or chickpeas.
4. Drizzle with gluten-free balsamic vinaigrette dressing.
5. Roll up the wrap and secure with a toothpick or wrap it in parchment paper for a gluten-free, on-the-go lunch.

4. Gluten-Free Mediterranean Bowl
Ingredients:
- Cooked quinoa (prepared in gluten-free vegetable broth)
- Cherry tomatoes, halved
- Cucumber, diced
- Kalamata olives, pitted and sliced
- Red onion, thinly sliced
- Fresh parsley, chopped
- Feta cheese (ensure it's gluten-free)
- Lemon-tahini dressing (gluten-free)

Instructions:
1. Cook quinoa in gluten-free vegetable broth according to package instructions.
2. In a bowl, combine cooked quinoa, halved cherry tomatoes, diced cucumber, sliced Kalamata olives, thinly sliced red onion, and chopped fresh parsley.
3. Crumble gluten-free feta cheese over the top.
4. Drizzle with gluten-free lemon-tahini dressing and toss to combine.
5. Portion the Mediterranean bowl into meal prep containers for a flavorful and satisfying gluten-free lunch or dinner.

5. Gluten-Free Berry Parfait
Ingredients:
- Gluten-free granola
- Greek yogurt (ensure it's gluten-free)
- Mixed berries (e.g., strawberries, blueberries, raspberries)
- Honey or maple syrup (gluten-free) for drizzling

Instructions:
1. In a glass or airtight container, layer gluten-free granola, Greek yogurt, and mixed berries.
2. Repeat the layers as desired.

3. Drizzle with honey or maple syrup for added sweetness.
4. Seal the parfait and store it in the refrigerator for a delightful gluten-free breakfast or snack option.

Gluten-free meal prep empowers you to embrace a delicious and safe dietary lifestyle while ensuring you have a variety of nutritious and flavorful meals at your fingertips. By maintaining a gluten-free kitchen, planning balanced meals, and using gluten-free substitutes, you can navigate your gluten-free journey with ease.

Keto-Friendly Meal Prep

The ketogenic (keto) diet has gained popularity for its potential to support weight loss, improve metabolic health, and boost mental clarity. It involves consuming a low-carbohydrate, high-fat diet, which forces the body to enter a state of ketosis, where it primarily burns fat for energy. Keto-friendly meal prep is a crucial aspect of successfully adhering to this dietary approach. In this chapter, we'll delve into the fundamentals of keto-friendly meal prep, explore its benefits, address potential challenges, and provide a collection of delectable keto recipes to elevate your culinary experience. The keto diet is built on a simple principle: drastically reduce carbohydrate intake and replace it with healthy fats and a moderate amount of protein. This change in macronutrient composition shifts the body's primary source of fuel from glucose (carbohydrates) to ketones (fat). Here's a breakdown of the macronutrient ratio typically followed in a keto diet:
- 70-75% Fat: Healthy fats like avocados, nuts, seeds, olive oil, and fatty cuts of meat are staples.
- 20-25% Protein: Moderate protein intake from sources such as poultry, fish, eggs, and tofu.
- 5-10% Carbohydrates: Limited carb consumption mainly from non-starchy vegetables and small portions of low-carb fruits.

Benefits of a Keto Diet
- Weight Loss: By shifting the body into ketosis, the keto diet encourages the burning of stored fat for energy, leading to weight loss.
- Improved Blood Sugar Control: Keto can help stabilize blood sugar levels, making it suitable for some individuals with type 2 diabetes.

- Enhanced Mental Clarity: Some people report increased mental focus and reduced brain fog when in ketosis.
- Appetite Control: The high-fat content and low-carb nature of keto meals can help reduce hunger and cravings.

Challenges of Keto Meal Prep

While keto offers numerous benefits, it can pose challenges in meal planning and preparation:
- Limited Food Choices: Eliminating many carb-rich foods can make meal planning seem restrictive.
- Increased Fat Intake: For some, consuming ample healthy fats can be an adjustment.
- Keto Flu: During the initial transition to ketosis, some people experience flu-like symptoms, including fatigue and headaches.
- Micronutrient Balance: Ensuring you get a variety of micronutrients can be challenging on a keto diet.

Keto-Friendly Meal Prep Essentials

Effective keto-friendly meal prep begins with thoughtful planning and the right kitchen tools and ingredients:
1. Plan Your Macros: Calculate your daily macronutrient needs (fat, protein, carbs) to create meals that align with your keto goals.
2. Kitchen Scale: Accurate portion control is essential in keto meal prep, so invest in a reliable kitchen scale.
3. Keto-Friendly Ingredients: Stock up on keto staples like avocados, nuts, seeds, olive oil, non-starchy vegetables (e.g., spinach, broccoli, cauliflower), and high-quality meats.
4. Meal Containers: Invest in meal prep containers to store your keto meals safely and conveniently.
5. Flavor Enhancers: Use keto-friendly flavor enhancers like herbs, spices, and sugar substitutes (e.g., erythritol, stevia) to keep your meals interesting.

Keto-Friendly Meal Prep Tips

1. Batch Cook Proteins: Prepare a variety of keto-friendly proteins (e.g., chicken, salmon, ground beef) and store them in portioned containers for easy meal assembly.
2. Roast Low-Carb Veggies: Roast vegetables like Brussels sprouts, asparagus, or zucchini with olive oil, salt, and pepper to have as sides or salad toppers throughout the week.

3. Pre-Portion Snacks: Portion out keto snacks like nuts, cheese cubes, or keto-friendly dips (e.g., guacamole) to curb cravings.
4. Make Keto Sauces: Prepare keto sauces and dressings in advance to add flavor to your meals without added carbs.
5. Plan for Breakfast: Plan keto breakfasts that don't require daily preparation, such as overnight chia seed pudding or crustless quiches.

Delectable Keto-Friendly Meal Prep Recipes

1. Keto-Friendly Chicken Caesar Salad
Ingredients:
- Grilled chicken breast, sliced
- Romaine lettuce, chopped
- Parmesan cheese, grated
- Sugar-free Caesar dressing

Instructions:
1. Toss sliced grilled chicken and chopped romaine lettuce together.
2. Sprinkle with grated Parmesan cheese.
3. Drizzle with sugar-free Caesar dressing.

2. Keto-Friendly Zucchini Noodles with Pesto
Ingredients:
- Zucchini noodles (zoodles)
- Homemade or store-bought keto-friendly pesto sauce
- Cherry tomatoes, halved
- Pine nuts, toasted

Instructions:
1. Sauté zucchini noodles in olive oil until tender.
2. Toss with keto-friendly pesto sauce.
3. Top with halved cherry tomatoes and toasted pine nuts.

3. Keto-Friendly Salmon with Lemon Butter Sauce
Ingredients:
- Salmon fillet
- Lemon juice
- Butter or ghee
- Fresh parsley, chopped

- Salt and pepper

Instructions:
1. Season salmon fillet with salt and pepper.
2. Sear in a hot skillet with butter or ghee until golden brown on both sides.
3. Finish by drizzling lemon juice and garnishing with chopped fresh parsley.

4. Keto-Friendly Cauliflower and Broccoli Mash
Ingredients:
- Cauliflower florets
- Broccoli florets
- Butter or ghee
- Garlic powder
- Salt and pepper

Instructions:
1. Steam cauliflower and broccoli until tender.
2. Blend with butter or ghee, garlic powder, salt, and pepper until smooth and creamy.

5. Keto-Friendly Chocolate Avocado Mousse
Ingredients:
- Ripe avocados
- Unsweetened cocoa powder
- Coconut milk
- Sugar-free sweetener (e.g., erythritol or stevia)
- Vanilla extract

Instructions:
1. Blend ripe avocados, unsweetened cocoa powder, coconut milk, sugar-free sweetener, and vanilla extract until smooth.
2. Chill in the refrigerator before serving.
Keto-friendly meal prep can be an exciting and effective way to embrace the benefits of the ketogenic diet. By understanding the principles of the keto diet, equipping your kitchen with the essentials, and following smart meal prep tips, you can create delicious, satisfying, and low-carb meals that align with your dietary goals.

Low-Carb Meal Prep

Low-carb diets have gained popularity for their potential to aid weight loss, improve blood sugar control, and increase overall metabolic health. These diets typically restrict the intake of carbohydrates, focusing on protein, healthy fats, and fiber-rich vegetables. Whether you're following a specific low-carb plan or simply looking to reduce your carb intake for health reasons, effective low-carb meal prep can be a game-changer in achieving your dietary goals. In this chapter, we'll delve into the essentials of low-carb meal prep, explore its benefits, address potential challenges, and provide a collection of mouthwatering low-carb recipes to elevate your culinary experience.

Understanding Low-Carb Diets

Low-carb diets come in various forms, including the ketogenic diet (very low carb, high fat), Atkins diet (gradually increasing carb intake in phases), and general low-carb diets (moderate carb restriction). The primary goal of these diets is to reduce carb consumption and encourage the body to burn fat for energy instead of relying on glucose from carbs.

Benefits of a Low-Carb Diet

- Weight Loss: By restricting carb intake, the body shifts to burning stored fat, leading to weight loss.
- Improved Blood Sugar Control: Low-carb diets can help stabilize blood sugar levels, making them suitable for individuals with type 2 diabetes.
- Reduced Cravings: Lower carb intake often results in reduced hunger and fewer sugar cravings.
- Enhanced Heart Health: Low-carb diets may improve heart health by lowering triglycerides and increasing HDL (good) cholesterol levels.

Challenges of Low-Carb Meal Prep

While low-carb diets offer many benefits, they can present certain challenges in meal planning and preparation:
- Reduced Carb Variety: Lowering carb intake may initially feel limiting in terms of food choices.

- Potential Keto Flu: Some individuals may experience flu-like symptoms when transitioning to very low-carb diets.
- Fiber Intake: Ensuring adequate fiber intake can be challenging, as many high-fiber foods are carb-rich.

Low-Carb Meal Prep Essentials

Effective low-carb meal prep starts with thoughtful planning and the right kitchen tools and ingredients:

1. Plan Your Macros: Calculate your daily macronutrient needs (carbs, protein, fats) to create meals that align with your low-carb goals.
2. Kitchen Scale: Use a kitchen scale for accurate portion control, especially when counting carbs.
3. Low-Carb Ingredients: Stock up on low-carb staples like lean proteins (chicken, turkey, tofu), non-starchy vegetables (spinach, broccoli, zucchini), healthy fats (avocado, olive oil), and low-carb sweeteners (erythritol, stevia).
4. Meal Containers: Invest in meal prep containers to store your low-carb meals safely and conveniently.
5. Flavor Enhancers: Use herbs, spices, and sugar substitutes (if needed) to add variety and taste to your low-carb meals.

Low-Carb Meal Prep Tips

1. Batch Cook Proteins: Prepare batches of lean proteins (e.g., grilled chicken, turkey meatballs) to use as the base for various low-carb meals.
2. Roast Low-Carb Veggies: Roast vegetables like Brussels sprouts, cauliflower, or asparagus with olive oil and your favorite seasonings to have as sides throughout the week.
3. Portion Snacks: Divide low-carb snacks like nuts, cheese cubes, or sliced veggies into individual portions to avoid overeating.
4. Homemade Dressings and Sauces: Create homemade low-carb salad dressings, marinades, and sauces to control ingredients and carb content.

Delectable Low-Carb Meal Prep Recipes

1. Low-Carb Chicken and Broccoli Stir-Fry

Ingredients:
- Chicken breast, thinly sliced
- Broccoli florets
- Low-sodium soy sauce or tamari

- Minced garlic
- Sesame oil
- Crushed red pepper flakes (optional)

Instructions:
1. In a hot skillet, stir-fry thinly sliced chicken breast until cooked through. Remove from the pan.
2. In the same skillet, add broccoli florets, minced garlic, and a splash of water. Steam until the broccoli is tender-crisp.
3. Return the cooked chicken to the skillet and add low-sodium soy sauce or tamari, sesame oil, and crushed red pepper flakes if desired.
4. Stir-fry until well combined. Portion into meal prep containers for a satisfying low-carb lunch or dinner.

2. Low-Carb Cauliflower and Spinach Soup
Ingredients:
- Cauliflower florets
- Fresh spinach
- Chicken or vegetable broth (low-sodium)
- Heavy cream (or coconut milk for a dairy-free option)
- Minced onion and garlic
- Olive oil
- Salt and pepper

Instructions:
1. In a large pot, sauté minced onion and garlic in olive oil until fragrant.
2. Add cauliflower florets and fresh spinach to the pot.
3. Pour in chicken or vegetable broth to cover the vegetables.
4. Simmer until the cauliflower is tender.
5. Blend the soup until smooth, then stir in heavy cream (or coconut milk).
6. Season with salt and pepper to taste. Divide into meal prep containers for a nourishing low-carb lunch.

3. Low-Carb Turkey and Avocado Lettuce Wraps
Ingredients:
- Ground turkey
- Romaine lettuce leaves

- Avocado slices
- Salsa
- Taco seasoning (low-carb)
- Shredded cheese (optional)

Instructions:
1. In a skillet, brown ground turkey and season with low-carb taco seasoning.
2. Lay out romaine lettuce leaves and fill with cooked turkey.
3. Top with avocado slices, salsa, and shredded cheese (if desired).
4. Roll up the lettuce leaves and secure with toothpicks. Store in meal prep containers for a low-carb, handheld meal.

4. Low-Carb Greek Salad with Grilled Chicken
Ingredients:
- Grilled chicken breast, sliced
- Cucumber, diced
- Cherry tomatoes, halved
- Red onion, thinly sliced
- Kalamata olives, pitted and sliced
- Feta cheese (optional)
- Greek dressing (low-carb)

Instructions:
1. Toss together grilled chicken breast, diced cucumber, halved cherry tomatoes, thinly sliced red onion, and sliced Kalamata olives.
2. If desired, add crumbled feta cheese.
3. Drizzle with low-carb Greek dressing and toss to combine.
4. Portion the Greek salad into meal prep containers for a refreshing low-carb lunch.

5. Low-Carb Berry Parfait
Ingredients:
- Greek yogurt (full-fat or low-fat)
- Mixed berries (e.g., strawberries, blueberries, raspberries)
- Low-carb granola or crushed nuts
- Sugar-free sweetener (optional)

Instructions:
1. In a glass or airtight container, layer Greek yogurt, mixed berries, and low-carb granola or crushed nuts.
2. If desired, add a sprinkle of sugar-free sweetener for extra sweetness.
3. Seal the parfait and store it in the refrigerator for a delightful low-carb breakfast or snack.

Low-carb meal prep can be both enjoyable and beneficial, allowing you to embrace a diet that supports your health and dietary goals. By understanding the principles of low-carb eating, equipping your kitchen with the essentials, and following smart meal prep tips, you can create delicious and satisfying low-carb meals that cater to your unique dietary needs. In the next chapter, we'll explore meal prep for individuals with specific health conditions, offering guidance and recipes tailored to their requirements.

Paleo Meal Prep

The Paleo diet, also known as the Paleolithic or caveman diet, takes inspiration from the eating habits of our ancient ancestors. This dietary approach emphasizes whole foods and encourages the avoidance of processed foods, grains, legumes, and dairy. By focusing on foods that were available to our ancestors during the Paleolithic era, proponents of the Paleo diet believe it can promote better health, support weight loss, and reduce the risk of modern-day chronic diseases. In this chapter, we'll explore the fundamentals of Paleo meal prep, examine the benefits, address potential challenges, and provide a collection of mouthwatering Paleo recipes to enhance your culinary journey.

Understanding the Paleo Diet
The Paleo diet centers on the consumption of foods that our pre-agricultural ancestors would have hunted, gathered, or foraged for. This includes:
- Lean meats: Such as beef, poultry, and game meats.
- Fish and seafood: Rich in essential fatty acids.
- Fruits: Including berries, apples, and other non-tropical fruits.
- Vegetables: Except for starchy vegetables like potatoes.
- Nuts and seeds: Such as almonds, walnuts, and flaxseeds.

- Healthy fats: From sources like avocados, olive oil, and coconut oil.

The Paleo diet excludes:
- Grains: Such as wheat, rice, and oats.
- Legumes: Including beans, lentils, and peanuts.
- Dairy: Except for some versions of the Paleo diet that allow limited dairy.
- Processed foods: Such as sugary snacks, processed meats, and artificial additives.

Benefits of the Paleo Diet
- Whole, Nutrient-Dense Foods: The Paleo diet emphasizes whole, unprocessed foods, providing essential vitamins and minerals.
- Weight Management: Many people find that the Paleo diet helps with weight loss due to its focus on satiating, nutrient-dense foods.
- Improved Blood Sugar Control: Reducing carb intake and avoiding sugar-laden foods can help stabilize blood sugar levels.
- Reduced Inflammation: Some individuals report a reduction in inflammatory markers when following a Paleo diet, which may benefit those with autoimmune conditions.

Challenges of Paleo Meal Prep
While the Paleo diet offers numerous benefits, it can present challenges in meal planning and preparation:
- Limited Carb Sources: The exclusion of grains and legumes can make it challenging to obtain adequate carbohydrates, particularly for athletes.
- Dairy Restrictions: Avoiding dairy may require finding suitable substitutes for milk, cheese, and yogurt.
- Planning and Variety: Meal planning can be time-consuming, and ensuring a variety of Paleo-friendly foods may require some effort.
- Social Situations: Dining out or attending social gatherings can be more challenging when following a strict Paleo diet.

Paleo Meal Prep Essentials
Effective Paleo meal prep starts with thoughtful planning and the right kitchen tools and ingredients:
1. Plan Your Paleo Meals: Create a meal plan that focuses on whole, Paleo-approved foods and incorporates variety.

2. Kitchen Essentials: Invest in tools like a good chef's knife, cutting board, and food storage containers to make meal prep easier.

3. Paleo Staples: Stock up on Paleo pantry staples like coconut flour, almond flour, coconut aminos (a Paleo-friendly soy sauce alternative), and a variety of herbs and spices.

4. Fresh Ingredients: Prioritize fresh fruits and vegetables, lean proteins, and healthy fats in your grocery shopping.

5. Batch Cooking: Prepare larger quantities of proteins and sides (e.g., roasted vegetables) to use throughout the week.

Paleo Meal Prep Tips

1. Prepare Proteins: Cook a batch of lean meats, such as chicken breasts, ground turkey, or salmon, to use as the base for various Paleo meals.

2. Roast Vegetables: Roast a variety of vegetables like broccoli, cauliflower, and Brussels sprouts with olive oil, salt, and herbs for easy side dishes.

3. Make Homemade Sauces: Create your Paleo-approved sauces and dressings using ingredients like olive oil, vinegar, herbs, and spices to add flavor to your meals.

4. Portion Snacks: Divide nuts, seeds, or Paleo-approved snacks like beef jerky into individual portions to avoid overeating.

Delectable Paleo Meal Prep Recipes

1. Paleo Grilled Chicken Salad

Ingredients:
- Grilled chicken breast, sliced
- Mixed greens
- Cherry tomatoes, halved
- Cucumber, sliced
- Red onion, thinly sliced
- Paleo-friendly vinaigrette dressing

Instructions:
1. Toss sliced grilled chicken breast, mixed greens, cherry tomatoes, sliced cucumber, and thinly sliced red onion in a large bowl.
2. Drizzle with Paleo-friendly vinaigrette dressing.

3. Portion into meal prep containers for a refreshing and satisfying Paleo salad.

2. Paleo-Friendly Beef and Vegetable Stir-Fry
Ingredients:
- Thinly sliced beef (e.g., sirloin or flank steak)
- Broccoli florets
- Red bell pepper, sliced
- Snow peas
- Paleo stir-fry sauce (made with coconut aminos, ginger, garlic, and honey or a sugar substitute)

Instructions:
1. In a hot skillet, stir-fry thinly sliced beef until cooked to your preferred level.
2. Remove the beef from the skillet.
3. In the same skillet, stir-fry broccoli florets, sliced red bell pepper, and snow peas until crisp-tender.
4. Return the cooked beef to the skillet and pour in the Paleo stir-fry sauce.
5. Stir-fry until well combined. Portion into meal prep containers for a flavorful Paleo lunch or dinner.

3. Paleo-Friendly Cauliflower Rice
Ingredients:
- Cauliflower florets
- Olive oil
- Minced garlic
- Fresh parsley, chopped
- Salt and pepper

Instructions:
1. Place cauliflower florets in a food processor and pulse until they resemble rice.
2. In a skillet, heat olive oil and sauté minced garlic until fragrant.
3. Add the cauliflower rice and sauté until tender.
4. Season with salt, pepper, and chopped fresh parsley.
5. Divide into meal prep containers for a versatile Paleo side dish.

4. Paleo-Friendly Guacamole and Veggie Sticks
Ingredients:
- Ripe avocados
- Lime juice
- Fresh cilantro, chopped
- Diced tomatoes
- Red onion, finely chopped
- Salt and pepper
- Sliced bell peppers, cucumber, and carrot sticks (for dipping)

Instructions:
1. In a bowl, mash ripe avocados and mix with lime juice.
2. Stir in chopped fresh cilantro, diced tomatoes, finely chopped red onion, salt, and pepper.
3. Serve with sliced bell peppers, cucumber, and carrot sticks for a Paleo-friendly snack.

5. Paleo-Friendly Dark Chocolate and Berry Parfait
Ingredients:
- Fresh mixed berries (e.g., strawberries, blueberries, raspberries)
- Full-fat coconut milk
- Dark chocolate chips (at least 70% cocoa)
- Unsweetened shredded coconut

Instructions:
1. In a glass or airtight container, layer fresh mixed berries and full-fat coconut milk.
2. Top with dark chocolate chips and unsweetened shredded coconut.
3. Seal the parfait and refrigerate for a delightful Paleo-friendly dessert or breakfast.

Paleo meal prep offers a unique culinary experience, allowing you to embrace whole, unprocessed foods while following the principles of the Paleolithic diet. By understanding the basics of the Paleo diet, equipping your kitchen with the essentials, and following smart meal prep tips, you can create delicious and wholesome Paleo meals that align with your dietary goals. In the next chapter, we'll explore meal prep for individuals with specific health conditions, offering guidance and recipes tailored to their unique needs.

Food Allergies and Intolerances

Food allergies and intolerances are common dietary concerns that require careful attention to meal preparation and ingredient choices. Individuals with food allergies experience an adverse immune response to specific proteins in foods, while those with food intolerances have difficulty digesting certain substances, often due to enzyme deficiencies. In this chapter, we'll explore the challenges posed by food allergies and intolerances, discuss strategies for safe meal prep, and provide a range of allergy-friendly and intolerance-friendly recipes to ensure everyone can enjoy delicious, safe meals. Food allergies are immune system reactions triggered by the ingestion of specific proteins in certain foods. Common food allergens include nuts, peanuts, milk, eggs, soy, wheat, fish, and shellfish. When someone with a food allergy consumes the allergenic food, their immune system perceives it as harmful and releases chemicals such as histamine, leading to symptoms that can range from mild hives to life-threatening anaphylaxis. Food intolerances, on the other hand, are typically non-immune responses to specific components of foods. Lactose intolerance, for example, results from a deficiency of the enzyme lactase, which is needed to digest lactose, a sugar found in milk and dairy products. Symptoms of food intolerances can include digestive discomfort, bloating, and diarrhea.

Challenges of Food Allergies and Intolerances
Managing food allergies and intolerances in meal preparation can be challenging due to the need to avoid specific ingredients and cross-contamination. Here are some common challenges:
- Ingredient Awareness: Individuals with allergies and intolerances must carefully read food labels and be aware of hidden sources of allergens or intolerant ingredients.
   Cross-Contamination: Preventing cross-contamination is crucial, as even trace amounts of allergenic foods can trigger reactions in those with allergies. This includes using separate utensils, cutting boards, and cookware.
- Limited Dining Out: Many individuals with food allergies or intolerances find it safer to prepare meals at home, as dining out can pose risks.

Safe Food Handling and Meal Prep

Safe meal prep for individuals with food allergies and intolerances requires attention to detail and careful planning:

1. Label Reading: Read food labels carefully to identify allergenic or intolerant ingredients.

2. Cross-Contamination Prevention: Use separate utensils and equipment for preparing allergen-free dishes. Clean surfaces thoroughly.

3. Communication: When cooking for someone with allergies or intolerances, communicate openly about their dietary needs and any specific restrictions.

4. Ingredient Substitutions: Familiarize yourself with allergy-friendly ingredient substitutions, such as almond flour for wheat flour or dairy-free milk alternatives.

Allergy-Friendly and Intolerance-Friendly Recipes.

Below are a few allergy-friendly and intolerance-friendly recipes that cater to common dietary restrictions:

1. Gluten-Free Chicken and Vegetable Stir-Fry

Ingredients:

- Sliced chicken breast
- Mixed vegetables (e.g., bell peppers, broccoli, carrots)
- Gluten-free tamari or soy sauce
- Minced garlic
- Sesame oil

Instructions:

1. In a hot skillet, stir-fry sliced chicken until cooked through. Remove from the skillet.

2. In the same skillet, stir-fry mixed vegetables with minced garlic and sesame oil until tender-crisp.

3. Return the cooked chicken to the skillet and drizzle with gluten-free tamari or soy sauce.

4. Stir-fry until well combined. Serve over gluten-free rice or cauliflower rice.

2. Dairy-Free Creamy Tomato Soup

Ingredients:

- Canned tomatoes
- Coconut milk (full-fat)

- Vegetable broth (low-sodium)
- Onion, diced
- Minced garlic
- Olive oil
- Fresh basil leaves (for garnish)

Instructions:
1. In a pot, sauté diced onion and minced garlic in olive oil until softened.
2. Add canned tomatoes, coconut milk, and vegetable broth to the pot.
3. Simmer until flavors meld and the soup is heated through.
4. Blend until smooth and creamy.
5. Garnish with fresh basil leaves before serving.

3. Nut-Free Energy Bites
Ingredients:
- Rolled oats (certified gluten-free if needed)
- Sunflower seed butter or tahini
- Honey or maple syrup
- Mini chocolate chips (allergen-free)
- Chia seeds

Instructions:
1. In a bowl, mix rolled oats, sunflower seed butter or tahini, honey or maple syrup, mini chocolate chips, and chia seeds until well combined.
2. Roll the mixture into bite-sized balls.
3. Refrigerate for at least 30 minutes before serving. These make for a nut-free and allergy-friendly snack.

4. Lactose-Free Potato Leek Soup
Ingredients:
- Potatoes, peeled and diced
- Leeks, cleaned and sliced
- Lactose-free milk (e.g., almond milk or lactose-free cow's milk)
- Vegetable broth (low-sodium)
- Olive oil
- Fresh thyme (for garnish)
- Salt and pepper

Instructions:
1. In a pot, sauté sliced leeks in olive oil until softened.
2. Add diced potatoes, vegetable broth, and lactose-free milk to the pot.
3. Simmer until the potatoes are tender.
4. Blend until smooth, season with salt and pepper, and garnish with fresh thyme.

5. Egg-Free Banana Pancakes
Ingredients:
- Ripe bananas, mashed
- Oat flour (certified gluten-free if needed)
- Baking powder
- Cinnamon
- Vanilla extract
- Non-dairy milk (e.g., almond milk)
- Cooking oil

Instructions:
1. In a bowl, mix mashed ripe bananas, oat flour, baking powder, cinnamon, vanilla extract, and non-dairy milk until you reach a pancake batter consistency.
2. Heat a skillet with cooking oil over medium heat.
3. Pour small portions of the batter onto the skillet to make pancakes.
4. Cook until bubbles form on the surface, then flip and cook until golden brown.
Managing food allergies and intolerances in meal preparation is essential for the health and well-being of those with dietary restrictions. By understanding the nature of food allergies and intolerances, practicing safe food handling, and exploring allergy-friendly and intolerance-friendly recipes, you can create delicious meals that cater to a wide range of dietary needs. In the following chapter, we'll delve into another dietary consideration—vegetarian and vegan meal prep—offering guidance and delectable recipes for plant-based meal enthusiasts.

Chapter 5
Staying on Track and Overcoming Challenges

Maintaining Motivation and Discipline

Maintaining motivation and discipline is an essential aspect of your journey towards successful weight loss and a healthier lifestyle. It's completely normal to experience moments of doubt or temporary setbacks, but with the right mindset and strategies, you can overcome these challenges and stay on course. Setting clear, achievable goals is the cornerstone of maintaining motivation and discipline. These goals give you a sense of direction and purpose. Start by setting both short-term and long-term goals. Short-term goals can be weekly or monthly targets, while long-term goals may span several months or even years. It's crucial to make these goals specific and realistic. Instead of merely saying, "I want to lose weight," be precise, like saying, "I aim to lose 10 pounds in the next three months." These clear objectives provide you with something concrete to work towards. Monitoring your progress is not only a helpful tool but also a motivating one. Keeping a journal or using a mobile app to record your meals, exercise routines, and changes in weight and body measurements allows you to visualize your journey. This visual representation of your hard work can serve as a powerful motivator and keep you disciplined. Celebrate every small victory, as they all contribute to your larger goals. Turning healthy behaviors into habits is a pivotal strategy in maintaining motivation and discipline. Repetition is key to forming habits, so the more you practice making nutritious choices and staying active, the easier it becomes. These habits gradually become an integral part of your daily life, making it less likely for you to deviate from your healthy path. Accountability can make a world of difference in your journey. Sharing your goals with a trusted friend or family member who can offer support and encouragement is invaluable. Alternatively, consider joining a weight loss group or finding a workout buddy. The sense of accountability keeps you committed to your goals, even when motivation takes a dip. Understand that setbacks are a natural part of any journey, including your path to a healthier lifestyle. Don't be too hard on yourself if you occasionally stray from your plan. Instead, view these setbacks as opportunities to learn and grow. Identify the factors that led to the setback and make necessary adjustments. Remember that every new day offers a fresh opportunity to make healthier choices. Visualization is a potent tool to maintain motivation. Imagine yourself successfully reaching your weight loss and fitness goals. Visualize how you'll look and feel when you achieve them. Use these mental images as a wellspring of inspiration. Additionally, employ positive affirmations to boost your self-confidence and maintain a positive attitude. Repeating phrases like "I am capable of reaching my goals" or "I am committed to a healthier lifestyle" can reinforce your determination.

Rewarding yourself for your hard work can provide an extra layer of motivation and discipline. Establish a reward system wherein you treat yourself when you hit specific milestones. Importantly, these rewards should not be food-based but rather something that brings you joy and reinforces your commitment to your goals. Consider treating yourself to a spa day, a new workout outfit, or a well-deserved weekend getaway. Don't hesitate to seek professional support when needed. Nutritionists, personal trainers, or mental health counselors can offer tailored guidance and strategies to address your unique needs and challenges. They can help you navigate obstacles and provide a fresh perspective on your journey. Lastly, shift your focus from short-term results to the long-term benefits of a healthier lifestyle. Maintaining motivation and discipline isn't just about reaching a specific number on the scale; it's about improving your overall health and well-being. Embrace the idea that your ultimate goal extends beyond mere numbers; it encompasses becoming a healthier and happier version of yourself. Stay motivated, stay disciplined, and embrace the transformation that awaits you on this incredible journey towards better health and vitality.

Handling Social Situations and Eating Out

This is a crucial skill for anyone looking to maintain a balanced and healthy lifestyle, as it allows you to enjoy social gatherings and restaurant experiences without compromising your dietary preferences or restrictions. Effective communication is at the heart of successfully navigating social situations. Informing your friends, family, and hosts about your dietary needs in advance is essential. By doing so, you create awareness and make it easier for them to accommodate your requirements. Consider offering to bring a dish that aligns with your dietary preferences when attending events or gatherings; most hosts appreciate the gesture and are accommodating when they understand your needs. Before dining out, research restaurants in your area that offer menu options aligned with your dietary preferences. Many restaurants now provide online menus, making it easier to identify suitable choices. Look for establishments that offer detailed menu descriptions or customizable dishes. Some even have separate menus for specific dietary needs, such as gluten-free or vegan options. When dining out, don't hesitate to ask questions and make special requests. Seek clarification from your server if a menu item isn't clear in terms of ingredients or preparation. Request modifications or substitutions to accommodate your dietary needs. Most restaurants are willing to accommodate reasonable requests, such as dressing on the side, omitting certain ingredients, or providing gluten-free alternatives. Managing portion sizes is another important aspect of dining out while staying true to your dietary goals. Restaurant portions are often larger than what you might typically consume at home. To avoid overindulging, consider sharing an entree with a dining companion or requesting a half-portion. Alternatively, ask for a to-go container when your meal is served and set aside a portion to take home before you start eating. Practicing mindful eating can be particularly beneficial when dining out. Mindful eating involves paying close attention to your food, savoring each bite, and eating slowly. It also means avoiding distractions like smartphones or TV screens at the table. By tuning into your body's hunger and fullness cues, you'll be less likely to overindulge and more likely to make healthier choices. Liquid calories, such as sugary cocktails, soft drinks, and alcoholic beverages, can significantly contribute to your overall calorie intake when dining out. Opt for water, unsweetened iced tea, or other low-calorie beverages to accompany your meal. If you choose to enjoy an alcoholic beverage, do so in moderation, as these drinks can add extra calories to your meal. In social situations where peer pressure or temptation is high, it's crucial to stay resilient and maintain your commitment to your dietary goals. Politely decline offers of food or drink that don't align with your preferences or restrictions. You can simply say, "No, thank you," or "I'm watching what I eat," without feeling the need to explain further. Building a supportive social circle can significantly impact your ability to stick to your dietary goals when faced with social situations. Seek out friends and acquaintances who respect and understand your dietary choices or restrictions. Sharing your journey with like-minded individuals can provide motivation and encouragement, making it easier to navigate social events. To simplify your dining out decisions, familiarize yourself with restaurant dishes or types of cuisine that align with your dietary preferences. Having a list of go-to options for various types of restaurants can streamline the decision-making process. For example, if you follow a low-carb diet, you might look for grilled protein and vegetable dishes on the menu. Special occasions like birthdays, holidays, and celebrations often involve indulgent meals and treats. Rather than feeling deprived, plan ahead for these occasions. Decide in advance what you'll indulge in and what you'll enjoy in moderation. By making intentional choices, you can participate in the festivities without derailing your progress. Lastly, remember to be kind to yourself throughout your journey. It's natural to occasionally deviate from your dietary goals, especially in social situations. Instead of dwelling on any perceived "mistakes," acknowledge them as learning experiences and opportunities for growth. Focus on your long-term progress and the positive choices you make daily. Handling social situations and eating out while staying committed to your dietary goals is an achievable skill that, with practice, allows you to maintain a balanced and enjoyable social life while adhering to a healthy diet.

Dealing with Plateaus

In the journey towards dietary improvements, weight management, or fitness goals, plateaus are a common occurrence that can often be frustrating. A plateau refers to a period where your progress seems to stall or slow down significantly, whether it's in terms of weight loss, dietary improvements, or fitness milestones. Despite your continued efforts, you find yourself at a standstill.

Plateaus manifest in various ways, and understanding why they happen and how to overcome them is essential for maintaining motivation and achieving long-term success. Weight loss plateaus are a familiar challenge for many on a weight management journey. It's the point where the number on the scale remains relatively stable for an extended period, despite your consistent dedication to losing weight. Dietary plateaus, on the other hand, may not always be as easily measurable but can still be a hindrance. These can manifest as a lack of noticeable changes in energy levels, mood, or overall well-being despite adhering to dietary adjustments. Fitness enthusiasts may encounter plateaus in terms of their strength, endurance, or the ability to reach new fitness milestones. Plateaus occur for a variety of reasons, and understanding these reasons is key to overcoming them effectively. One significant factor is metabolic adaptation. Your body is highly adaptive and strives to maintain balance. As you lose weight or make dietary improvements, your metabolism may slow down as a way to conserve energy. This slowdown can make it more challenging to continue seeing progress. Another reason for plateaus is reaching calorie equilibrium. Your calorie intake and calorie expenditure reach a point where they balance each other out. This equilibrium results in weight maintenance rather than further loss. Habituation is another factor, where your body and mind become accustomed to the changes you've made over time. The initial excitement and results may diminish, leading to a plateau. Stress, hormonal fluctuations, and sleep disturbances can further complicate the picture by affecting your body's ability to make progress. Overcoming plateaus requires a combination of strategies and a patient, determined mindset. One approach is to reevaluate your goals. Are they realistic, achievable, and sustainable? Adjusting your goals if necessary can provide fresh motivation and clarity. Reviewing your current plan is also crucial. Whether it's your meal plan, exercise routine, or dietary improvements, identify areas where positive changes or variety can be introduced. Tracking your progress through detailed records of your meals, workouts, and body measurements can help you pinpoint patterns or areas needing adjustments. Changing your routine can also be beneficial, as your body may have adapted to your current practices. Experiment with new workouts, alter your meal timings, or explore different types of foods to keep things fresh and challenging.

Shifting your focus away from the scale, especially during a weight loss plateau, can be liberating. Celebrate non-scale victories like increased energy levels, better sleep, or enhanced strength. Managing stress is another critical aspect of overcoming plateaus. High stress levels can hinder progress, so implement stress-management techniques such as meditation, deep breathing exercises, or yoga to help your body relax. Adequate sleep and recovery are equally important. They play a significant role in overall well-being and weight management. Ensure you're getting enough rest to support your body's functions. Seek professional guidance if you find it challenging to overcome a plateau on your own. A registered dietitian, personal trainer, or healthcare professional can offer tailored advice and adjustments to your plan. Practice patience throughout the process. Plateaus are temporary setbacks, not permanent roadblocks. Stay positive and motivated, surround yourself with a supportive community, or seek out inspirational stories to keep you focused on your goals. By implementing these strategies and maintaining a determined mindset, you can effectively navigate plateaus and continue progressing towards your health and dietary objectives. Remember that plateaus are opportunities for growth and learning, and with perseverance, you'll emerge stronger and more resilient on your journey.

Celebrating Your Weight Loss Successes

Celebrating your weight loss successes is a vital part of your journey towards improved health and well-being. It's essential to acknowledge and commemorate your achievements, no matter how small or significant they may seem. Celebrations not only boost your morale and motivation but also reinforce the positive behaviors and habits that have led to your success. In this chapter, we'll explore the importance of celebrating your weight loss successes and provide tips on how to do so effectively. First and foremost, it's crucial to recognize that every step forward, no matter how modest, is a significant accomplishment. Whether you've shed a few pounds or reached a major milestone in your weight loss journey, each success is a testament to your determination and hard work. It's easy to get caught up in the ultimate goal, but celebrating your progress along the way is essential for maintaining a positive mindset and sustaining your motivation. One of the most powerful aspects of celebrating your weight loss successes is the positive reinforcement it provides. When you acknowledge your achievements, whether by sharing them with friends and family, treating yourself to a small reward, or simply giving yourself a pat on the back, you're reinforcing the behaviors and choices that led to your success. This positive feedback loop can help solidify the healthy habits you've developed and encourage you to continue making them a part of your daily life. Moreover, celebrating your successes can boost your self-esteem and confidence. Weight loss journeys often come with moments of doubt and self-criticism. By taking the time to celebrate your achievements, you remind yourself of your capabilities and the progress you've made. This self-affirmation can be a powerful tool for overcoming self-doubt and building a more positive self-image.

Celebrations need not be extravagant or costly. In fact, the most effective celebrations are often simple and heartfelt. Here are some tips on how to celebrate your weight loss successes:

1. Set Milestones: Break your weight loss journey into smaller, manageable milestones. Celebrate each milestone reached, whether it's losing a certain number of pounds, fitting into a smaller clothing size, or achieving a fitness goal.

2. Share Your Success: Don't hesitate to share your achievements with friends and family who have supported you along the way. Their encouragement and celebration of your successes can be incredibly motivating.

3. Non-Food Rewards: Avoid celebrating with food rewards, as this can undermine your progress. Instead, opt for non-food rewards like buying yourself a new outfit, treating yourself to a spa day, or planning a weekend getaway.

4. Create a Success Journal: Keep a journal where you document your successes, big and small. Write down how you felt when you achieved a goal and the positive changes you've experienced. Periodically revisit your journal to remind yourself of your progress.

5. Photographic Evidence: Take progress photos throughout your journey. Comparing these photos over time can be a powerful visual representation of your success and a great source of motivation.

6. Celebrate With Friends: Consider organizing a celebration with friends or fellow weight loss companions who understand the significance of your achievements. Share your stories, accomplishments, and challenges, creating a supportive and encouraging atmosphere.

7. Give Back: Use your successes as an opportunity to give back. Volunteer your time or donate to a charity that aligns with your values. Helping others can be a meaningful way to celebrate your own accomplishments.

8. Set New Goals: After celebrating a success, set new goals to continue your journey. This ensures that you always have something to work towards and look forward to.

9. Practice Self-Compassion: Be kind to yourself throughout your journey. Celebrate your successes, but also acknowledge that setbacks and challenges are a natural part of the process. Treat yourself with the same compassion you would offer to a friend.

10. Maintain Balance: While celebrating successes is essential, it's equally important to maintain balance. Avoid excessive or self-indulgent celebrations that may undo your hard work. Instead, opt for celebrations that align with your health and wellness goals.

Celebrating your weight loss successes is a fundamental aspect of your journey towards improved health and well-being. It reinforces positive behaviors, boosts self-esteem and confidence, and provides motivation to continue making healthy choices. Whether you're celebrating small milestones or significant achievements, the act of celebrating itself is a powerful tool for maintaining a positive mindset and sustaining your progress. So, take the time to acknowledge and commemorate your successes, and remember that every step forward is a reason to celebrate.

Conclusion

Final Thoughts and Words of Encouragement

As you approach the conclusion of your journey towards improved health, dietary changes, or weight management, it's essential to reflect on your achievements, acknowledge your growth, and find inspiration in the progress you've made. This final chapter serves as a source of encouragement and a reminder that your journey is ongoing, filled with endless possibilities for continued success. Throughout this journey, you've demonstrated resilience, determination, and a commitment to your well-being. You've made choices that align with your goals, whether it's shedding pounds, adopting a healthier lifestyle, or embracing a dietary regimen. You've overcome obstacles, learned valuable lessons, and experienced personal growth. It's important to recognize and celebrate these achievements, no matter how small they may seem. Embrace the idea that your journey is not defined by a specific destination but by the continuous effort and dedication you invest in yourself. You've laid the foundation for lasting change, and your accomplishments are a testament to your inner strength. Every step you've taken, every healthy choice you've made, and every obstacle you've surmounted has brought you closer to a happier, healthier version of yourself. Remember that setbacks and plateaus are a natural part of any transformative journey. They do not define your progress or your potential for success. Instead, they offer valuable opportunities for learning and growth. Approach setbacks with resilience and a willingness to adapt. Use them as stepping stones to propel you forward, and never lose sight of your ultimate goals. As you move forward, set new goals and challenges for yourself. Whether you're aiming to achieve new fitness milestones, explore different aspects of your chosen dietary path, or maintain your current level of success, the journey continues. Keep your motivation high by envisioning the future you desire and the positive impact it will have on your life. Surround yourself with a supportive community of friends, family, or like-minded individuals who understand and appreciate your journey. Share your successes and challenges, seek advice when needed, and offer your support to others who may be on a similar path. The power of a supportive community cannot be underestimated, as it can provide motivation, encouragement, and a sense of belonging. Maintain a mindset of self-compassion throughout your journey. Understand that perfection is not the goal; progress is. Be kind to yourself in moments of difficulty or self-doubt. Treat yourself with the same compassion you would offer to a friend facing similar challenges. Remember that setbacks do not define your worth or your ability to achieve your goals. Celebrate every success, no matter how small or seemingly insignificant. Acknowledge the effort and dedication you've put into your journey and use each achievement as motivation to keep moving forward. Reward yourself in ways that align with your health and wellness goals, and find joy in the progress you've made. In your journey towards improved health, dietary changes, or weight management, you hold the power to shape your future. You have the ability to continue making choices that support your well-being and happiness. Your journey is a testament to your strength, resilience, and commitment to personal growth. As you move forward, carry with you the lessons you've learned, the successes you've celebrated, and the support of your community. Embrace the challenges that lie ahead as opportunities for further growth and transformation. Trust in your ability to navigate this journey with wisdom and determination. In closing, remember that your journey is a lifelong pursuit of health, well-being, and self-improvement. It is filled with moments of triumph and moments of struggle, but each experience contributes to your growth and resilience. Be encouraged by your progress, find inspiration in your goals, and continue moving forward with confidence. Your journey is a testament to your strength, and the possibilities for a healthier, happier you are limitless.